ADVANCE PRAISE

"Dr. Tom Guttuso has hit a home run for the Parkinson's community with his new book, *The Promise of Lithium*. It's written in plain, easy-to-understand English so that everyone can follow his conclusions, and at the same time, Dr. Guttuso anticipates the questions from real live patients like me! This book will be part of my active collection on my desk."

—Jack Quinn, former US Congressman, current Parkinson's disease patient, and Michael J Fox Foundation board member

"Through page after stunning page of *The Promise of Lithium*, Dr. Guttuso amps up the urgency and cranks up hope for people with Parkinson's and Alzheimer's. The author's bold assertions, backed by hundreds of sources, will have the readers rooting for him and lithium. The neuroprotective promise will spark conversation and kick up some dust in the Parkinson's community."

—Larry Gifford, President of PD Avengers and Parkinson's disease patient

"Dr. Tom Guttuso is a respected neurologist who now has proven himself to be a highly talented writer. In his book, he talks in detail about scientific issues related to the causes of Alzheimer's and Parkinson's and the potential role of lithium as a treatment, yet he manages to do so in a highly engaging and thoughtful way that anyone can understand. If you want to understand the data on lithium and its potential promise for Alzheimer's and Parkinson's, there is no better source than this book."

—David K. Simon, MD, PhD; Professor of Neurology at Beth Israel Deaconess Medical Center and Harvard Medical School

"Dr. Tom Guttuso is a wonderful neurologist, a caring clinician, and a keen observer. In this book, he explores the potential therapeutic benefits of lithium for treating two debilitating diseases that affect one out of every ten Americans over sixty-five and provides truly novel insights into them."

—Ray Dorsey, MD; Professor of Neurology at the University of Rochester and co-author of *Ending Parkinson's Disease*

THE

PROMISE

OF

LITHIUM

THOMAS GUTTUSO, JR., MD

THE

PROMISE

OF

LITHIUM

HOW AN OVER-THE-COUNTER
SUPPLEMENT MAY PREVENT AND SLOW
ALZHEIMER'S AND PARKINSON'S DISEASE

To my wife,
who tries her best to appear interested
when I'm talking science.

DISCLAIMER: *The information in this book is not intended to and should not be used as a substitute for a doctor's medical advice. A licensed physician should be consulted regarding all health matters as well as any medical symptoms that are occurring. Over-the-counter supplements should be taken under the supervision of a health care professional.*

THE PROMISE OF LITHIUM
How an Over-the-Counter Supplement May Prevent and Slow Alzheimer's and Parkinson's Disease

ISBN	978-1-5445-3545-6	*Hardcover*
	978-1-5445-2954-7	*Paperback*
	978-1-5445-3544-9	*Ebook*

CONTENTS

EVERY DAY THAT PASSES IS A DAY BRAIN CELLS VANISH

FOR OVER 20 YEARS, my patients have asked me the same question: "Why have there not been any breakthroughs in the treatment of Alzheimer's or Parkinson's disease?" My answer has always been the same: "These diseases are complicated, and unfortunately, it's been very challenging to find a treatment that can stop or even slow their progression." My patients' looks of disappointment and frustration have become very familiar and disheartening to me. Patients bring in articles of "highly promising" or "exciting" experimental treatments for me to read and ask when they could try one of these. They don't realize that virtually all of these studies have been done on isolated brain cells living in petri dishes or in animals. I explain that dozens of drugs have shown excellent results in animal studies, typically in mice or rats, but then have completely failed in human studies. How can this be? Is it that our animal models are not accurately representing what happens in humans with Alzheimer's and Parkinson's and are leading us down unfruitful paths? Is it because humans' brains are much more complicated than rodents' brains? When I look at all of the experimental treatments that I have initially been excited about and later been disappointed in, sometimes I wonder if we have made any progress at all.

All of that changed when a Parkinson's patient of mine named Ted (not his real name) and his wife came in for a routine follow-up office visit in 2014 and told me something that sent me down a rabbit hole of information gathering after which my outlook and hope on the treatment of both Parkinson's disease (PD) and Alzheimer's disease (AD) were radically transformed. Ted and his wife told me that day that one of Ted's most severe and difficult-to-treat PD symptoms called motor fluctuations almost fully resolved soon after Ted's psychiatrist put him on a low dose of lithium medication to treat his concomitant bipolar disorder. This came as a complete surprise to me not only because I had never heard of lithium being beneficial for PD but because Ted's motor fluctuations were so severe and disabling, he was close to needing brain surgery to get them under control. Fascinated by Ted's story, I started reading every medical journal article I could find on how lithium could possibly be responsible for such a dramatic improvement in Ted's symptoms. What I learned surprised me even more than what Ted and his wife told me that day in 2014. What I learned and subsequently discovered is what this book is all about.

You may believe that there is nothing that can be done to prevent or slow the progression of AD or PD. This is not true.

What is true is that there is nothing *proven* to do these things. Nevertheless, if you are one of the 45 million people in the world living with AD or PD, you probably want to know if there is anything that *may* slow the progression of these diseases. Adhering to healthy lifestyle habits such as exercising every day and maintaining a Mediterranean diet may help to slow AD and PD progression and definitely will help to prevent heart disease and stroke. This book will not discuss the potential benefits of exercise and a healthy diet. This book will describe a treatment that has far more convincing and comprehensive evidence than any other treatment, supporting its ability to prevent and slow the progression of AD and PD. Even better, this treatment is an all-natural, over-the-counter (OTC) supplement available to everyone.

Sound too good to be true? You will soon understand that it's not. For over 20 years there have been multiple studies in laboratories, animal models of AD and PD and, most importantly, in *human patients* with AD and PD that show this all-natural treatment to protect brain cells and potentially prevent and slow AD and PD. This treatment is not new. In fact, it's so old that it even predates the formation of the earth. It's one of the original elements formed at the genesis of the universe. This treatment is lithium.

There is a saying in neurology: TIME IS BRAIN. This statement is typically used for treating patients with an acute stroke when time is of the essence in order to administer a clot-busting drug that can greatly reduce the stroke's damage to the brain and improve a patient's level of function. For stroke patients, there is a 4.5-hour window from the onset of the stroke symptoms until the clot buster needs to be injected. After 4.5 hours, with very few exceptions, it's too late. The window has closed.

With AD and PD, the window is literally decades long.

But don't let this fool you into complacency thinking you have decades to treat these diseases. AD and PD patients should have nearly the same sense of urgency as stroke patients. Why? Because just like with stroke, TIME IS BRAIN. Every day brain cells are dying in AD and PD patients, slowly leading to mounting disability and impaired independence. If there is a treatment that could slow down this process, why wait? The sooner it is delivered, the more brain cells can be saved. In AD and PD, saving brain cells is the name of the game. Once the cells have died, there is no bringing them back. They are gone forever.

You may not realize this now, but AD and PD progress relentlessly over many years to the point where patients with either disease eventually end up in an unfortunately dark place: repeated falls, confused, and in need of significant care or nursing home placement. Fortunately, it takes an average of about 10 years to get to this stage. But, make no mistake, everyone with AD or PD will eventually reach this place if they live long enough. Not only do AD and PD slowly rob people of their quality of life, but they are killers. Most studies cite AD as the sixth leading cause of death in the United States; however, there is evidence that this is a gross underestimation of AD's lethality. When accounting for the medical problems caused by progressed AD that lead to death, AD then becomes the third leading cause of death in the US just behind heart attacks and cancer.[1] In terms of the annual price tag of treating and caring for AD patients, it dwarfs that of heart attacks and cancer.[2] With the aging of the world's population, AD and PD are rapidly growing in prevalence.

If time is brain in AD and PD, now is the time for you to read this book. Every day that passes is a day brain cells vanish.

This book will not tell you that lithium is a miracle cure for these diseases. I will tell you now that it is not. What this book will do is empower you with knowledge. Finding a way to prevent and slow down AD and PD has been an unsolvable puzzle for scientists for decades. In this book, you will see how many pieces of this puzzle come together to form a picture of hope. Hope is an essential state of mind for anyone diagnosed with these diseases or, for that matter, with any disease. Hope is also necessary for anyone who loves someone with these diseases. Hope itself without any other intervention has tremendous healing abilities. I can guarantee that after reading this book you will have hope. Not false hope or unfounded hype, but true hope that progress is being made in our fight to prevent and slow AD and PD. In particular, after reading this book you will likely share in my belief and the belief of many other scientific researchers that low-dose daily lithium supplementation may prevent and slow the progression of AD and PD and help preserve these patients' futures. You will see how over 200 pieces of evidence from peer-reviewed medical journal publications referenced throughout this book come together to form this picture of hope.

History has taught us that some of the most important discoveries in medicine were made by accident. The critical ingredient necessary for turning an accidental discovery into a proven treatment that can benefit patients is an inquisitive researcher who champions the cause. There are hundreds of such discoveries in medical history. Two of the earliest and most consequential examples are when James Lind proved in 1747 that eating citrus fruit cured a gruesome disease called scurvy; and when Edward Jenner proved in 1796 that intentionally giving someone a mild infection with cowpox protected them from contracting an often-lethal infection of smallpox.[3] In each of these instances, the initial observations from which these therapies stemmed actually occurred several or even hundreds of years earlier. The discoveries were based on unexpected observations; the proof was based on research.

I have been fortunate to have made four such accidental discoveries over my career and, more importantly, to have also performed the research on the first three to prove that these treatments provided benefits to patients. The first discovery and subsequent research study publication led to a novel, nonhormonal medication treatment for hot flashes in postmenopausal women and a US patent licensed by Pfizer.[4] The second discovery eventually led to a grant from the National Institutes of Health to support research on the third discovery demonstrating this same medication to also be the very first treatment to significantly improve the severe nausea, vomiting, and malnutrition of early pregnancy called hyperemesis gravidarum, the condition that afflicted Princess Kate Middleton and landed her in the hospital when she was pregnant with her first baby, George.[5] The fourth discovery became the origin of this book.

Over the past 23 years, my research has resulted in 34 original publications in peer-reviewed medical journals and many presentations at medical meetings. However, educating the non-medical world on this information is an entirely different matter. This is the purpose of this book: to educate and inform AD and PD patients and caregivers as well as doctors in easy-to-understand language that does not require an MD or PhD to appreciate. I have had the education and training in medical school, neurology residency, and experimental therapeutics fellowship; experience performing both basic science animal research and human clinical trial research and of turning accidental discoveries into real-world treatments that have enabled me to bring this information to you. More importantly, when I hear a patient like Ted tell me he feels remarkably better after starting a new treatment, that makes me motivated: motivated to move the needle, advance medical knowledge, and, hopefully, improve patients' lives through research.

This book will likely ruffle some feathers. That is fine. For serious diseases like AD and PD that have no proven ways to prevent or slow them down, the more valid and easy-to-understand information available for patients to absorb, the better. This is your life. This is your brain. This is your future.

This book will take a deep dive, explaining the known causes of AD and PD, the targets in the brain that need to be engaged in order to effectively prevent and slow these diseases, and the evidence dating back to 1959 showing why lithium makes such good sense in these functions. (For those who want to take an even deeper dive, all of the facts cited are referenced at the end of the book and can be Googled.) I'll explain why there's a holdup in advancing the development of lithium for AD and PD and exactly what types of research need to be performed to hopefully someday prove that lithium can slow the progressive worsening of symptoms in AD and PD. Finally, I'll conclude with all of the practical information one will need in order to make an informed decision on whether or not to take over-the-counter (OTC) lithium supplementation while waiting for this research to be performed; the pros and cons of the two OTC lithium formulations available; and a review of the available data one will need in choosing an appropriate dosage.

You will then truly appreciate how the pieces of this puzzle come together to form a stunning picture of hope.

CHAPTER 1

THE BRAIN'S BERMUDA TRIANGLE

IN THE WORLD'S QUEST to find an effective way to prevent and slow the progression of Alzheimer's disease (AD) and Parkinson's disease (PD), you will be surprised to discover that there is extensive evidence that an element hidden in one of the most dangerous consumer products readily available behind the cashier at virtually every gas station may accomplish these vaulted feats. This dangerous product is cigarettes.

Sounds crazy, but it's true. Of course, no sane doctor would ever recommend that an AD or PD patient start smoking. But what if this specific element that is hidden in tobacco was safe and could be isolated, purified, and provided in a capsule that is available as an over-the-counter (OTC) supplement? This would offer AD and PD patients the opportunity to take this element every day without exposing themselves to all of the other dangerous compounds in tobacco. Fortunately, this has already been done. The element is lithium.

If you have AD or PD, you have probably performed at least one Google search looking for a treatment that could possibly slow down the progression of your disease and preserve your current level of function for many years into the future. For AD patients, you likely have learned that in 2021 a therapy called aducanumab was approved by the US Food and Drug Administration (FDA) for slowing the progression of AD. Yet, there is still much uncertainty whether or not aducanumab is actually effective despite it being FDA-approved. In addition, this drug can cause brain swelling and brain bleeding. For these reasons, many private insurance companies and Medicare have either refused to pay for aducanumab or have greatly restricted its coverage. If you have PD, your Google search has revealed that there currently are no FDA-approved treatments to slow the progression of PD over time. There are only PD treatments, such as levodopa, that can mask your symptoms but that become less effective over time as the disease progresses.

In short, if you have AD or PD, you have likely come to realize that your disease symptoms will relentlessly progress over time, and there is not much that your doctor can do to change this reality.

However, this is not the full reality. There are some things that you can be doing right now such as daily aerobic exercise or adhering to a diet high in vegetables and low in red meats, dairy, and refined sugars that may help slow down your disease. While there is evidence to support these interventions, you will soon come to appreciate that there is far more extensive and high-quality evidence that daily lithium supplementation may prevent and slow AD and PD. In order to understand and appreciate this important news, it will greatly help for you to first understand our current knowledge about what causes AD and PD.

What Causes AD and PD?

Upon being diagnosed with AD or PD, the first question patients usually have is, "How did I get this?" The answer to this question is not very satisfying for patients. About 93% of AD and PD cases are due to some combination of environmental exposures in a person genetically at risk. Probably less than 7% of AD or PD cases are caused by a specific gene inherited from one or both parents. Thus, most patients with AD or PD have no family members with either of these diseases. Regardless of whatever combination of environmental and genetic factors trigger the start of these diseases, the destructive processes that cause the progressive death of brain cells and the consequent worsening of symptoms over time are nearly identical in AD and PD. Identifying and understanding these destructive processes allows researchers to identify and study treatments to potentially slow AD and PD.

What are these destructive processes? They are toxic sticky proteins, inflammation, and oxidative stress: "The Brain's Bermuda Triangle" (Figure 1). Uncovering why these destructive processes start in patients with AD and PD will take some detective work. So put on your Sherlock Holmes hat, and let's get to it.

FIGURE 1:
THE BRAIN'S
BERMUDA TRIANGLE

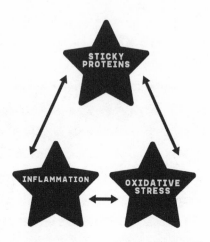

Just like when a detective is attempting to solve a murder, the key is to go to the scene of the crime. Let's take an example of a person found dead in a park due to a bullet wound. It would be pretty hard for the detective to determine who shot him just based on this initial information. However, if the detective uses a special chemical that lights up trace amounts of blood and sprays it on the ground around the body, it shows there is a track of blood traversing the park across the street and into a warehouse where the deceased person worked. Where the blood trail stops, the detective finds a bullet in the wall that matches the bullet in the deceased. With some investigation, the detective discovers that the bullet was shot from the gun registered to this person's boss. Furthermore, the detective discovers that the deceased was about to blow the whistle on illegal activities that the boss was committing, and the boss had found out the day prior that the deceased was going to tell the local authorities. The detective now has the murder location, the murder weapon, and the motive. Case closed.

Solving a mystery is no different in neurology. Localization in the brain is not only key to making an accurate diagnosis but also for identifying the cause(s) of the condition. So where is the scene of the crime at the very start of AD and PD? In other words, where in the nervous system does AD and PD damage begin? Identification of these locations will likely provide strong clues about the causes of these diseases, which will help identify new treatments.

Similar to the special spray the detective used to locate the blood drops in the park, scientists have used a special stain on brain slices from deceased AD and PD patients to reveal where their characteristic sticky proteins first appear. These studies have revealed that AD starts in a part of the brain called the locus coeruleus (pronounced soe-roo-lee-us), and PD starts in two places in the nervous system: the olfactory bulb and the myenteric plexus that innervates the gut.[6] I know you have probably never heard these terms before. That's okay. You will soon understand these terms and, furthermore, understand why they are important for putting the pieces of the puzzle together to help solve this mystery.

For AD, there are two types of sticky proteins in the brain that mark the disease process: beta-amyloid plaques that accumulate/aggregate on the outside of brain cells and tau tangles that aggregate on the inside of brain cells. For PD, there is only one sticky protein called alpha-synuclein that aggregates on the inside of brain cells. It is the sticky proteins inside cells that best correspond to where brain cells die and what consequent symptoms a patient with AD or PD experience.[7] Thus, when looking for the scene of the crime in AD and PD, scientists agree it is best to examine where tau tangles and alpha-synuclein, respectively, first appear.

Not only do these sticky proteins mark the locations where AD and PD start, but they also mark what new locations become involved as AD and PD progress over time. That's because these sticky proteins do not stay put in one location. They spread. And they don't spread to random locations. They spread in a very predictable fashion along established brain pathways just like water flowing predictably down a river. These brain pathways can be thought of like tiny streams in the brain. As the sticky proteins accumulate on the banks of a stream at one location, they eventually travel into the stream's current and spread downstream to the location at the end of the stream. After arriving at their new downstream location, they take up residence and multiply. It is the progressive spreading and multiplication of sticky proteins in concert with the two other destructive processes of the Brain's Bermuda Triangle, inflammation and oxidative stress, that lead to the progressive death of brain cells in connected brain regions and the consequent progressive worsening of symptoms in AD and PD over time.

We learned above that AD starts in the locus coeruleus and PD starts in the olfactory bulb and the myenteric plexus. Why do AD and PD start in these locations, and what does that tell us about the causes of AD and PD? If we can find clues about why these locations are so important for the initiation of AD and PD, perhaps we can then find treatments to prevent and slow the

Brain's Bermuda Triangle of destruction and, thus, prevent and slow AD and PD.

Let's start with AD.

Alzheimer's Disease (AD)

As stated above, tau tangles first appear in the locus coeruleus in AD before spreading to other connected locations.[8] The first two locations where tau tangles spread from the locus coeruleus are the olfactory bulb, which processes our sense of smell, and a group of brain areas involved with short-term memory and cognition.[9] As a result, the earliest symptoms that can be detected in an AD patient are a decreased sense of smell and impaired short-term memory abilities.[10] But years before these symptoms begin, tau tangles have taken up residence in the locus coeruleus. What is so special about the locus coeruleus that would make it particularly vulnerable and represent the scene of the crime of AD initiation?

A very unique feature of the locus coeruleus is that it has a highly extensive network of connections to the brain's blood vessels/vasculature. The magnitude of connections that the locus coeruleus has with brain vasculature dwarfs than of any other brain site.[11] This massive network of connections between the locus coeruleus and the brain's vasculature establishes a strong bidirectional communication pathway where the brain's vasculature can "talk to" the locus coeruleus and vice versa. What could be going on in the brain's vasculature that would communicate to the locus coeruleus to begin the formation of tau tangles? The answer lies in the Brain's Bermuda Triangle. As depicted by the bidirectional arrows in Figure 1, both inflammation and oxidative stress can trigger the formation of sticky proteins such as tau tangles.[12] But what could initially cause inflammation and oxidative stress in the brain's vasculature that would then trigger the formation of sticky tau tangles in the locus coeruleus? To find the answer, we simply need to look at the most prominent risk factors for developing AD.

As you can see from Table 1, the most prominent risk factors for developing AD are the same factors that increase a person's risk for developing heart disease and strokes; namely, high blood pressure, diabetes, high cholesterol, and smoking.[13]

Table 1: Risk Factors for Alzheimer's Disease (AD)

Vascular Risk Factor	Increased Risk for AD
High Blood Pressure	25%[14]
Diabetes	57%[15]
High Cholesterol (LDL)	30%[16]
Smoking	72%[17]

LDL: low-density lipoprotein; cohort study data reported when available.[18]

This makes perfect sense because all of these risk factors are well known to cause inflammation and oxidative stress in blood vessels, leading to a build-up of plaque on the vessel walls, the narrowing of blood vessels, and eventually a full blood clot/

occlusion.[19] If the occlusion occurs in one of the blood vessels supplying blood to the heart muscle, a heart attack occurs. If the occlusion occurs in one of the blood vessels supplying blood to the brain, a stroke occurs. Most people think of strokes as causing dramatic neurological symptoms such as paralysis on one side of the body or an inability to speak. These are symptoms for big strokes that stem from the occlusion of a big blood vessel in the brain. However, very small strokes can occur in many parts of the brain that cause no immediate symptoms at all. These are called silent strokes from "small vessel disease." Because the vascular risk factors of high blood pressure, diabetes, high cholesterol, and smoking are risk factors for both AD and strokes, it should come as no surprise that progressive strokes, both small and large, are associated with a much greater risk for dementia in general and AD specifically.[20]

At this point we should clarify some language. Dementia is a general term referring to any condition causing the progressive decline of memory and other cognitive abilities like communicating, reasoning, calculating, or navigating resulting in problems with everyday activities. All types of dementia, including AD, are diagnosed based on these clinical symptoms. AD is one particular type of dementia. In fact, AD is the most common type of dementia accounting for about 70% of all cases. Other less common types of dementia like frontotemporal dementia and Lewy body dementia are also caused by the Brain's Bermuda Triangle, which shows not only the general importance of these destructive processes but also how valuable it would be to identify therapies that could effectively quell each tip of the Brain's Bermuda Triangle (Figure 1).

FIGURE 2A:
THE ALZHEIMER'S HOUSE
WITH A LEAKY ROOF
BEFORE DIAGNOSIS

● – Tiny Strokes
IO = Inflammation + Oxidative Stress
T – Tau

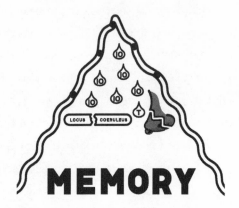

FIGURE 2B:
THE ALZHEIMER'S HOUSE
WITH A LEAKY ROOF
AT DIAGNOSIS

● – Tiny Strokes
IO = Inflammation + Oxidative Stress
T – Tau

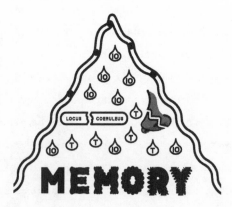

This progressive spreading of brain cell destruction in AD is depicted in Figures 2A and 2B: "The Alzheimer's House with a Leaky Roof." Inflammation and oxidative stress begin in the brain's blood vessels (depicted in the roof of the house) where they can cause small blood vessel occlusions and strokes. The inflammation and oxidative stress in the brain's blood vessels then flow downstream to the locus coeruleus, where they trigger tau tangles to first take root. After tau tangles have taken root here, they multiply and eventually travel downstream from the locus coeruleus to a few other connected regions including the olfactory bulb (causing inflammation, oxidative stress, brain cell damage, and a consequent decline in a person's sense of smell) and several brain sites important for cognition (causing impaired memory and other cognitive abilities). Due to this predictable cascade of brain damage among connected locations, it can be appreciated that an impaired sense of smell alone or in combination with mild short-term memory impairment can be the very first clinical symptoms in a person destined to develop AD in the near future (Figure 2A).[21] Because TIME IS BRAIN, as discussed in the Introduction, the best time to act and initiate a "neuroprotective treatment" would be as early as possible in the course of AD, which would be as soon as a decreased sense of smell and/or abnormal degree of forgetfulness can first be detected.

And what constitutes a "neuroprotective treatment" for AD or PD? Once again, the answer lies in Figure 1. An effective neuroprotective treatment for AD or PD would be one that effectively quells all three points of the Brain's Bermuda Triangle: sticky proteins, inflammation, and oxidative stress. As these are the three most important targets that need to be engaged and quelled in AD and PD, we need to understand a bit more about each of them to solve this mystery, just like the detective needed to identify the shooter's motive to solve the murder mystery.

Inflammation

Inflammation is a natural process that occurs when there is an injury in the body. For example, if you sprain your ankle when stepping off of a curb, your ankle will swell, hurt, and maybe turn red. These inflammatory reactions occur due to the flood of chemicals called cytokines into the site of the ankle injury. Cytokines are released by white blood cells that are constantly circulating in your blood stream patrolling your whole body for injury or infection. When white blood cells detect a problem, they release cytokines to alert other white blood cells to accumulate at the site of the problem and activate healing mechanisms. In this acute setting, inflammation is a good thing to help heal your sprained ankle. However, chronic inflammation that occurs over long periods of time can destroy healthy tissue including the brain.

There is a particular type of white blood cell that resides in the brain called microglia. As sticky proteins such as tau tangles and alpha-synuclein aggregates accumulate inside brain cells (aka neurons), microglia detect this as a problem and release cytokines. Because the sticky proteins are tenacious and resistant to being cleared, microglia perceive this as a continuous problem leading to further microglial activation, persistent release of cytokines, and progressive damage to all of the neurons in the vicinity.

In other words, acute inflammation is protective but chronic inflammation is destructive. If we could calm down microglial activation and the release of cytokines, we could reduce chronic inflammation and the consequent collateral damage to neurons as well as inflammation-induced formation of sticky proteins and oxidative stress (Figure 1).[22] The bottom line is that reducing microglial activation is likely an essential step for preventing and slowing AD and PD.

Sticky Proteins

Assuming chronic inflammation and/or oxidative stress have already triggered the formation of sticky proteins inside brain cells, like in patients already diagnosed with AD or PD, is it possible to clear them out? Because these sticky proteins are located inside brain cells, an effective therapy would first need to be able to gain access to this location and second be able to engage some process inside brain cells to increase the clearance and/or reduce the formation of sticky proteins. A perfect therapy would have easy access into brain cells and robustly engage intracellular machinery that is already on site and known to have these effects. For sticky proteins to form, first the proteins need to be produced (aka protein synthesis) and then the proteins need to be made sticky (aka protein modification). The main type of protein modification that makes the AD protein tau sticky is called phosphorylation. Thus, reducing the phosphorylation of tau would be beneficial to reduce the stickiness of the tau protein. On the clearance side, brain cells already have little garbage collectors on site called lysosomes whose job is to dispose of proteins that are no longer beneficial to the brain cell. Excessive sticky protein clutter inside brain cells can spoil the cell just like excessive kitchen clutter can spoil a meal. A small amount of clutter is easily manageable. However, overwhelming clutter will make it impossible to find untainted ingredients and prepare and cook an edible meal. If the kitchen can't produce meals, it's pretty useless. If a brain cell is full of sticky protein clutter, it also becomes useless and eventually will die. The take-home message is this: protein clutter is a killer.

Advanced age is the main risk factor for developing AD and PD, which have average ages of onset of about 72 and 62 years old, respectively.[23] It's likely not a coincidence that lysosomal function progressively declines with age and that both AD and PD have significantly more lysosomal dysfunction than expected for their ages at diagnosis.[24] Furthermore, accumulated sticky proteins themselves can cause lysosomal dysfunction leading to a vicious cycle where lysosomal dysfunction leads to sticky protein accumulation, which then leads to more lysosomal dysfunction.[25] With the garbage collectors out sick, the cellular clutter mounts. If there was a therapy that could improve lysosomal function, the accumulation of sticky proteins could be slowed or halted in AD and PD.

Now let's talk about the third destructive process in the Brain's Bermuda Triangle.

Oxidative Stress

Oxidative stress occurs when a type of chemical called free radicals is produced and causes immediate damage to adjacent tissue. There are many causes of free radical formation including microglial activation[26]; however, a primary source is from an organelle called mitochondria that are found in almost all cells in the body including brain cells. Mitochondria are like microscopic power plants that transform the energy trapped in the food that we eat into a chemical called ATP needed by cells to survive. Without a constant supply of ATP, all cells will die. As a byproduct of the process of producing ATP, mitochondria also produce some free radicals much like a nuclear power plant generates some radioactive waste in the process of generating electricity. If mitochondria are healthy, very limited amounts of free radicals are produced. Small amounts of free radicals can either be neutralized by natural antioxidants inside and around mitochondria or result in a limited and sustainable amount of damage to surrounding tissue. However, if mitochondria are sick or damaged, they will start spilling excessive amounts of free radicals like a damaged nuclear power plant spilling excess radioactive waste into the surrounding land.[27] Large amounts of free radicals will overwhelm the cell's natural antioxidants and cause increasing and unsustainable damage to surrounding tissue. This unchecked oxidative stress can then trigger the formation of sticky proteins like tau tangles and alpha-synuclein aggregates as well as trigger microglia to release cytokines leading to increased inflammation.[28] Thus, therapies that can preserve or improve mitochondrial health and function can reduce oxidative stress.

I hope that it is now clear that each of these three damaging processes (spreading and multiplying sticky proteins, chronic inflammation, and oxidative stress) can trigger the other two, thereby forming the Brain's Bermuda Triangle (Figure 1). Due to this vicious triangle of self-perpetuating destruction, you can now appreciate why all three of these processes would need to be effectively targeted and quelled by a treatment in order to successfully prevent and/or slow the progression of AD or PD. If only one or two processes are successfully targeted, the other unchecked process(es) will continue to wreak havoc inside the brain, eventually overwhelming the treatment's actions and likely eliminating any benefit to the AD or PD patient.

The bottom line is that if we want to make a difference in the prognosis of AD and PD, we need to successfully quell all three damaging processes either with multiple different treatments or with one treatment that engages all three targets: microglia, lysosomes, and mitochondria.

If you think that's a tall task, there's yet another task that any AD or PD treatment needs to accomplish. It must be able to penetrate two formidable barriers: the blood-brain barrier and the brain cell wall.

Almost all animals that have a brain also have a blood-brain barrier, which keeps most harmful substances that are eaten or inhaled confined to the bloodstream and out of the brain. In this way, the blood-brain barrier protects brain cells and brain function so that the animal can retain its ability to protect itself in the circumstance that it has inhaled or eaten something harmful. When designing a drug to treat any brain disease including AD and PD, the drug needs to have very specific qualities in order to cross the blood-brain barrier. Assuming a drug is actually able to cross this barrier, it still needs to cross the neuronal or microglial cell wall to enter the brain cell, and it must cross at a high enough concentration to effectively engage all three points of the Brain's Bermuda Triangle without causing intolerable side effects to the

AD or PD patient. Hopefully you are now starting to appreciate why finding treatments to slow AD and PD progression has been such a big challenge for researchers.

Just like in AD, the Brain's Bermuda Triangle is also responsible for the progressive brain cell death and progressive worsening of symptoms in PD. The only difference is that the sticky protein in PD is alpha-synuclein instead of tau and these sticky alpha-synuclein proteins start in different parts of the nervous system than where tau tangles start in AD.

Parkinson's Disease (PD)

PD is diagnosed when a patient has at least two of three signs on a neurological examination: a tremor (rhythmic shaking) usually in one hand that occurs when the hand is at rest in their lap, slowness of movement, and muscle stiffness. If a person has two or all three of these signs, they will likely qualify for a diagnosis of PD. However, just like in AD, the disease does not start in the part of the brain responsible for the symptoms from which the diagnosis is made. In fact, one of the two sites where the PD sticky alpha-synuclein aggregates starts isn't even in the brain! It's in a part of the nervous system that innervates the gut called the myenteric plexus.[29] The resulting dysfunction in the gut from alpha-synuclein–induced damage is believed to be what causes the frequent occurrence of constipation in patients years before they are diagnosed with PD.[30] The other site where sticky alpha-synuclein aggregates first appear is in the olfactory bulb resulting in a decreased sense of smell,[31] which typically predates the PD diagnosis by many years just like in AD.[32] A final symptom that often portends PD in the near future is a strange sleep disorder when people act out their dreams while sleeping, called REM sleep behavior disorder, which is also a result of alpha-synuclein aggregates appearing in connected brain pathways (Figure 3A).[33]

It is important to note that the sticky alpha-synuclein aggregates in PD start in areas of the nervous system that are most extensively exposed to the outside environment, which consists of the air we breathe and the food we eat. This is important because some particular environmental exposures including the air pollutant nitrogen dioxide, certain pesticides and toxins, and influenza viral infection are major risks for developing PD (see Table 2). These risk factors make sense because it is known that pesticides, nitrogen dioxide, and viral infections all cause inflammation and oxidative stress in exposed tissue.[34]

Table 2: Risk Factors for PD

Environmental Exposure	Increased Risk for PD
Pesticides	70%[35]
Nitrogen Dioxide Pollutant	41%[36]
Infection with Influenza	73%[37]

Cohort study data reported when available.[38]

Inhaled air pollution, pesticides, or influenza virus have direct access to the brain's olfactory bulb, located just above the nose, while pesticides and other toxins that we eat have direct access to the gut's myenteric plexus. These environmental insults causing inflammation and oxidative stress can then trigger the formation of alpha-synuclein aggregates in the olfactory bulb and myenteric plexus and start the disease process of PD. Over many subsequent years, these alpha-synuclein aggregates flow downstream along established nervous system pathways until they reach a part of the brain called the substantia nigra that produces an important brain chemical/neurotransmitter called dopamine. Brain dopamine levels are very important for allowing us to move in a smooth and coordinated fashion. As the alpha-synuclein aggregates accumulate in the dopamine substantia nigra neurons, they trigger increasing levels of inflammation and oxidative stress (see Figure 1), which leads to the progressive death of these dopamine neurons. Once about 50% have died, patients will start to develop the characteristic motor signs of PD (hand tremors, muscle stiffness, and slowness of movement), leading to a diagnosis of PD (Figure 3B). Patients remember that day of diagnosis as the day that their PD started. However, as you can now appreciate, the initial disease process of PD started many years or perhaps even decades before an actual diagnosis of PD. As previously mentioned, in addition to a decreased sense of smell or constipation, another symptom PD patients can get years before they are diagnosed with PD is the strange sleep disorder when people act out their dreams while sleeping, called REM sleep behavior disorder (Figure 3A).

FIGURE 3A:
THE PARKINSON'S HOUSE
WITH A LEAKY ROOF

BEFORE DIAGNOSIS

— Influenza Virus
IO — Inflammation + Oxidative Stress
A — Alpha-Synuclein

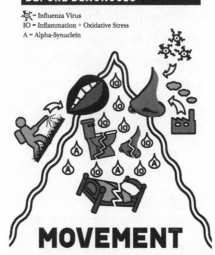

MOVEMENT

FIGURE 3B:
THE PARKINSON'S HOUSE
WITH A LEAKY ROOF

AT DIAGNOSIS

— Influenza Virus
IO — Inflammation + Oxidative Stress
A — Alpha-Synuclein

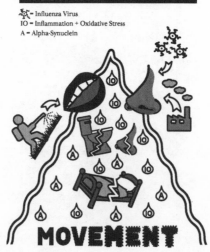

MOVEMENT

Because TIME IS BRAIN in both PD and AD, the best time to act and initiate a neuroprotective treatment would be as early as possible in the course of PD, which would be as soon as a decreased sense of smell, moderate constipation, and/or REM sleep behavior disorder can first be detected.

Not only is it important to note in Table 2 that exposure to environmental factors are prominent risks for PD, but it's equally as important to note that the vascular risk factors of high blood pressure, high cholesterol, smoking, and the consequent increase in strokes that are all prominent risks for AD are all *not* risk factors for PD (Table 3). In fact, there is evidence that PD patients actually have a reduced amount of small vessel strokes compared to age-matched people without PD, which is the complete opposite of what is seen in AD.[39]

Table 3: Comparison of Associations Between Vascular Risk Factors and Risks for Developing AD versus PD

Vascular Risk Factor	Increased Risk for AD	Increased Risk for PD
High Blood Pressure	25%[40]	Negligible[41]
Diabetes	57%[42]	34%[43]
High Cholesterol (LDL)	30%[44]	Negligible[45]
Smoking	72%[46]	-77%[47]

Cohort study data reported when available.[48]

What's Going On with Smoking?

If you have been paying attention, you hopefully noticed something very strange in Table 3. It is no surprise that smoking is associated with a large increased risk for developing AD because many of the compounds in tobacco are toxic to blood vessels and cause inflammation and oxidative stress in the blood vessel wall.[49] As previously reviewed, factors that cause blood vessel inflammation or oxidative stress—such as high blood pressure, diabetes, and high cholesterol—can trigger the start of AD in the brain's locus coeruleus (Figure 2A). That would explain why smoking is associated with a large 72% increased risk for AD. But why is smoking also associated with an even larger 77% *reduced risk* for developing PD (Table 3)? Your first thought may be that this was just a fluke finding from one or two studies. After all, smoking is one of the worst things a person can do for their health. As surprising as it is, this was far from a fluke finding.

Starting with the first report in 1959,[50] there have been over 60 independent studies involving different populations from different countries all showing very consistent results: smoking is associated with a greatly reduced risk for developing PD.[51] In addition, people exposed to secondhand smoke also have a reduced risk for developing PD. This argues against the possibility that some other quality inherent in PD patients, such as having a risk-averse personality leading PD patients not to smoke, accounts for the reduced risk of PD in smokers.[52] One particularly interesting study looked to see if the rates of PD changed between women and men in the second half of the twentieth century during the time when rates of smoking increased in women and decreased in men.[53] In this natural history-type of clinical trial, it was shown that the risk of PD decreased in women and increased in men in the second half versus first half of the twentieth century, which is exactly what would be expected if there was a neuroprotective element in tobacco that protected against PD. Furthermore, this study confirmed that smoking was having real health effects because, in addition to the results on PD rates, men and women had reduced and increased rates of lung cancer, respectively, in the second half versus first half of the twentieth century. We know that toxic carcinogens in tobacco cause lung cancer in smokers. Thus, the observation that lung cancer and PD rates historically moved in opposite directions in men and women associated with their disparate changes in smoking rates argues strongly that there is a neuroprotective element in tobacco that is protecting against PD. In line with the results of this study, the rapidly rising rates of PD currently seen in industrialized countries has been theorized to be due, in part, to the continued decreasing rates of smoking in the population.[54]

The whole body of observational study evidence suggests that smoking actually causes a decreased risk for PD due to there being a neuroprotective element in tobacco; however, there still is a chance that genetic factors in smokers or PD patients are influencing this consistent observation of reduced PD risk in smokers. A powerful method for controlling for the potential influence of genetics is to examine sets of identical twins and see if a twin who smokes is less likely to develop PD than a twin who does not smoke. Because twins have virtually identical genetic make-ups and very similar lifestyles, any differences found between the two twins in disease occurrence are highly likely due to differences in the environmental exposure (i.e., smoking) and not some unknown genetic factor. These twin studies have actually been performed, and indeed, this is exactly what was found: the twin who smoked had a significantly reduced risk of PD compared to their identical twin who did not smoke.[55] Finally, autopsy studies have shown that smokers have significantly less brain alpha-synuclein aggregates than nonsmokers, which further supports the conclusion that some element in tobacco counteracts the underlying disease process in PD and protects against this disease.[56]

The challenge with identifying the neuroprotective compound in tobacco is that tobacco contains thousands of compounds, any one or combination of which could be neuroprotective.[57] Despite this fact, the compound in tobacco that has received the most attention toward this end is nicotine. Because nicotine demonstrated some benefit in PD animal models, nicotine was then studied in some small clinical trials in PD patients.[58] These initial small clinical trials showed conflicting results. Therefore, in order to answer the question of whether nicotine slowed PD symptoms more definitively, the Michael J. Fox Foundation funded the largest PD nicotine trial that has ever been performed, the NIC-PD trial.

In this study, PD patients at multiple medical centers in the United States and Germany who had recently been diagnosed with PD and were not taking most PD medications were randomly assigned to either a nicotine patch or an identically appearing patch that had no nicotine (i.e., a placebo patch) for one year.[59] Patients' PD symptoms were evaluated in a double-blind fashion (i.e., neither the patients nor the doctors knew what each patient was receiving) after 52 weeks of patch treatment and again after the patches were removed for eight weeks.

The hope was that the PD patients receiving nicotine patches would have less severe PD symptoms compared to the patients receiving placebo patches at both the 52-week and 60-week time points, which would show that nicotine was slowing the worsening of symptoms in PD possibly by protecting against the progressive loss of brain cells. Surprisingly, this study showed the exact opposite results! PD patients receiving nicotine patches did *worse* than patients receiving placebo patches at both time points.[60] Talk about a disappointment. How could it be that all of this evidence showing that smokers have a reduced risk of PD failed so dramatically when nicotine was put to the test in a clinical trial?

There are several possible explanations for these findings, but the most glaring is that the researchers picked the wrong compound in tobacco to study. Even though nicotine showed some benefit in PD animal models, these models have proven to mislead us time and time again. It is clear that these animal models do not fully reflect what is happening in PD patients' brains and, as a result, have repeatedly misled the scientific community. As evidence, one only needs to look at the dozens of treatments that have shown great promise in PD animal models that have subsequently completely flopped when put to the test in human PD patients.[61]

Suffice it to say that it would be immensely valuable in our quest to prevent and slow both PD and AD if some promising *human data* were available to bolster promising animal data on a particular treatment. One big problem is that the vast majority of drug development effort comes from pharmaceutical companies that focus on developing completely new drugs for which they can receive patent protection. With a patent in hand, the company can then recoup their research and development costs and turn a profit if the drug eventually gets FDA-approved. This is understandable and usually beneficial to patients because it supercharges the whole drug development process.

However, the necessity of patent-protection to justify pharmaceutical company investment eliminates any such investments into developing old drugs for a completely different disease (aka "drug repurposing"). That leaves foundations like the Michael J. Fox Foundation or the Alzheimer's Association and government funding agencies like the National Institutes of Health (NIH) to fund research on such "repurposed" treatments. There are a few big problems with this process. First, foundations and government funding agencies have very limited funds available to grant to researchers, which makes it highly competitive to secure funding. As a result, many excellent ideas with great potential are left unfunded. Potential cures fall by the wayside perhaps for decades. Sometimes these great ideas get funded and tested, but very often they don't. The other big problem is that even when ideas do get funded, the whole process takes a very long time. For example, it took eight years from when funding was first sought for the NIC-PD trial to when the study was complete and the results were presented. If nicotine was a new drug under patent by a pharmaceutical company, this timeline would have been shortened to about two years or less.

Fortunately, the NIC-PD trial was funded, and the results were definitive: nicotine is not the neuroprotective element in tobacco. If it's not nicotine, then is there another element in tobacco that is known to be neuroprotective? Most importantly, is there any *human* evidence that this element in tobacco may prevent or slow the progression of symptoms in AD and PD patients? The answer is yes! It is lithium.

CHAPTER 2

WHY LITHIUM?

BECAUSE PRESCRIPTION LITHIUM THERAPY is highly effective for treating bipolar disorder,[62] a condition where people cycle between periods of irrational euphoria and depression, researchers in India had a hypothesis that people who consumed foods with a high lithium content would have lower rates of bipolar disorder. In order to test this hypothesis, they first needed to assess the lithium content in 60 popular Indian foods, spices, and beverages. Fortunately, these researchers also tested the lithium content in Indian tobacco because chewing tobacco is quite popular in India. The results published in 1980 showed that out of all 60 items tested, the highest levels of lithium were found in *tobacco*.[63] In fact, the lithium levels in tobacco were over 18 times higher than the second-highest item tested: black-eyed peas. The researchers devoted very little attention in their article to this unexpected finding. But I sure took notice. And now you understand why I did.

You may be wondering right now why it took so long for this connection to be made. After all, it has been repeatedly observed since 1959 that smokers have a greatly reduced risk of developing

PD, repeatedly shown since 1999 that lithium has a multitude of neuroprotective actions (to be detailed later in this chapter), and shown in 1980 that tobacco has very high levels of lithium. How could it be that it took until 2019 for these three simple facts to get connected with the theory that lithium was the potential, elusive neuroprotective element in tobacco protecting against PD?[64]

The Connection Between Smoking, Lithium, and PD

As a practicing movement disorder neurologist for 22 years, I care for many PD patients. As mentioned in the Introduction, it wasn't until 2014 that I became interested in lithium completely by accident when a PD patient of mine named Ted (not his real name) and his wife told me that one of Ted's most severe and difficult-to-treat PD symptoms called motor fluctuations almost fully resolved soon after Ted's psychiatrist put him on a low dose of lithium to treat his concomitant bipolar disorder. The more I talked to Ted and his wife that day, the more I was intrigued. I had never heard of lithium being beneficial for PD. I had only heard about lithium toxicity, when too high of a dose was used, sometimes actually causing Parkinson's-type symptoms. But Ted and his wife were reporting the exact opposite: that Ted's PD symptoms had greatly *improved* since starting lithium. Because they were both so pleased with how well Ted was doing, I hit the computer to perform a literature search. What I eventually discovered was a true eureka moment.

The first thing I found was that in 1982 researchers at Duke University Medical Center had reported the same finding that

Ted and his wife had observed: a big reduction in motor fluctuations in five of six PD patients treated with lithium.[65] However, just two years later in 1984, this same research group at Duke reported that all five of these patients initially experiencing improvements in motor fluctuations eventually developed severe jerky, squirming movements called dyskinesias within one to seven months of starting lithium, and most needed to discontinue lithium.[66] Over the following 30 years, there was no further research performed on lithium's ability to reduce motor fluctuations in PD.

When Ted and his wife came into my office that day, Ted had been taking lithium for five months and had no signs of worsening dyskinesias or any other side effects. How could it be, I wondered, that the Duke researchers found that 100% of their PD patients on lithium for one to seven months experienced severe dyskinesias, and Ted had not?

There is a quote from a sixteenth-century Swiss physician named Paracelsus that is as true today as it was back then: "The dose makes the poison."

Virtually everything in nature, if ingested in excess, will cause side effects and sometimes even death. This is true of over-the-counter medications like Tylenol and aspirin, prescription medications, and even water. This is especially true of lithium. Too high of a dose of lithium can definitely cause side effects and can even be lethal. But too low of a dose will be ineffective, at least for treating the only condition for which lithium is FDA-approved, bipolar disorder. The correct lithium dose for an individual patient is determined by measuring the lithium level in the bloodstream. For almost all patients with bipolar disorder, this correct or "therapeutic" blood serum lithium level falls between 0.6–1.2 millimoles per liter (mmol/L). Lithium levels below 0.6 mmol/L usually are ineffective, while levels greater than 1.2 mmol/L usually cause bothersome and sometimes disabling side effects. Psychiatrists' years of experience have shown that a serum lithium level of 0.6–1.2 mmol/L is the therapeutic sweet spot for treating bipolar disorder.

In 1982, the Duke researchers assumed that PD patients would have the same serum lithium sweet spot as bipolar patients in order to improve their motor fluctuations. Thus, lithium dosing was adjusted so that the average serum lithium level among the five PD patients in this Duke study was 0.8 mmol/L. When Ted and his wife came to my office that day in 2014, Ted's serum lithium level was only 0.4 mmol/L.

Could it be, I wondered, that PD patients only required half the lithium dose of bipolar patients in order to achieve benefit to their motor fluctuations without the side effect of increased dyskinesias? I followed Ted closely over the next six months, and he continued to have almost no motor fluctuations and never developed worsening dyskinesias at a lithium blood level that stayed around 0.4 mmol/L. I eventually tried this "low-dose" lithium therapy in several more of my PD patients and observed the same very promising results that I had observed in Ted.[67] Even more exciting than the benefits I was seeing in my PD patients' motor fluctuations was what I was learning about a completely different and much more urgent potential use of lithium: as a treatment to prevent and slow the progressive death of brain cells in AD and PD.

After scouring through medical literature, I came to realize there were literally hundreds of published studies showing that lithium can protect brain cells in laboratory cell cultures, in animal models of AD and PD, and most importantly, *in humans* with AD. After taking a step back and really thinking about lithium, it dawned upon me that lithium is far more than a drug. Lithium is the third element in the Periodic Table of Elements and, as such, is part of our earth. This clearly was a quality about lithium that distinguished it from all other drugs previously studied to treat AD or PD. Understanding that lithium was part of the earth and most living matter, I wondered if lithium was found in higher concentrations in certain foods just like the elements potassium and calcium are found in high concentrations in bananas and milk, respectively. And if lithium concentrations were high in certain foods, I wondered if there was any evidence that ingestion of these foods was linked with lower rates of AD or PD.

What I found on page three of my Google search almost knocked me off my chair. It was the 1980 study from India showing sky-high levels of lithium in tobacco. Eureka! The connection was made between smoking, lithium, and PD.

Now, what to do with this discovery? After all, the notion that lithium was the key neuroprotective element in tobacco was still just a theory. I thought that the first order of business was confirming that there were similarly high lithium concentrations in popular US brands of cigarette tobacco as was found in Indian tobacco. My research group at the University at Buffalo performed these analyses and showed that lithium levels in tobacco from Marlboro and Camel cigarettes were as high or higher than those in Indian tobacco.[68] I theorized that the tobacco plant, for whatever reason, must concentrate lithium absorbed from the soil into its leaves. This seemed a bit strange to me. Why would the tobacco plant do this?

It turns out, the tobacco plant doesn't just concentrate lithium in its leaves; it concentrates all the metals it absorbs from the soil into its leaves. I didn't realize it at the time, but the chemical properties of lithium classify it as a metal. Lithium is actually the lightest metal on earth. The tobacco plant, *Nicotiana tabacum*, is exceptionally efficient at absorbing all metals from the soil— even much heavier metals than lithium such as cadmium, thallium, and lead—and concentrating them in its leaves. On the other hand, most other nontobacco plants retain the majority of such absorbed metals in their roots.[69] In fact, the tobacco plant is so efficient at absorbing heavy metals that there is an agricultural practice of planting tobacco in contaminated fields in order to remove toxic metals like cadmium and lead from the soil in preparation for cultivating vegetable plants—a process called "phytoextraction."[70] Interestingly, the tobacco leaf concentrates the light metal lithium at least ten times greater than it does the heavy metal cadmium. One cigarette contains about 0.0018 mg and 0.017 mg of cadmium and lithium, respectively.[71] Considering the molecular weight of cadmium is 16 times greater than lithium, this means that tobacco concentrates lithium elements 150 times greater than cadmium elements. Because the leaf is the part of the tobacco plant that is smoked in cigarettes, smokers are exposed to high amounts of all of these metals from the inhaled smoke.[72] Many of these metals, especially cadmium, cause inflammation and oxidative stress and are carcinogenic (i.e., cancer-causing).[73] These metals are efficiently absorbed through the lungs and into the bloodstream and are also present in exhaled smoke. This is reflected in the higher levels of cadmium and lead in the bloodstream of smokers as well as in the hair of children exposed to secondhand smoke.[74]

Although it has not been formally studied to date, it is highly likely that the lightest metal on earth that is highly concentrated in the tobacco leaf (i.e., lithium) will also be found in high levels in the bloodstream of smokers and those exposed to secondhand smoke just as are the heavier metals of cadmium and lead. Because there are 20 cigarettes in a pack, a pack-per-day smoker would inhale about 0.34 mg of lithium a day (0.017 mg/cigarette times 20). As you will read in the next chapter, a daily lithium dosage of 0.3 mg was shown to significantly slow cognitive decline *in patients with AD*.[75] These findings imply that very small daily dosages of lithium may be able to slow AD and PD. Because "the dose makes the poison," as Paracelsus stated, a smaller effective dose of any medication or all-natural supplement, like lithium, would translate into a reduced likelihood for side effects in the patient. If a dosage of only 0.3 mg/day of lithium was shown to effectively slow AD and/or PD, that would represent an ideal therapy as this low of a dosage is much, much lower than the dosage known to possibly cause lithium-induced side effects.

In summary, my new theory was that inhaled lithium from smoking would not only be absorbed through the lungs and into the bloodstreams and brains of smokers leading to a decreased risk of PD, but also that lithium would be present in exhaled smoke accounting for the significant PD risk reduction observed in those exposed to secondhand smoke.[76] At first blush, this theory appeared to be a perfect present for PD patients, complete with a cute little bow. However, there was one problem.

How Could Smoking Cause AD but Prevent PD?

If you've been paying attention, you should be asking yourself a question right now. If inhaled lithium from smoking is responsible for the decreased risk of PD in smokers, and lithium is generally neuroprotective, then why don't smokers also have a decreased risk for AD? In fact, how can we explain why smokers have a 72% *increased* risk for AD (Tables 1 and 3, Chapter 1) if lithium in tobacco is neuroprotective?[77] Although there is currently no definitive answer to this question, I propose that it's simply a matter of real estate.

Neurology is very much like the real estate market: the most important feature is location, location, location. As we reviewed earlier, AD and PD start in very different locations in the nervous system: AD starts in the locus coeruleus, and PD starts in the olfactory bulb and the myenteric plexus. It is possible that smoking causes such profound inflammation and oxidative stress in the brain's blood vessels and consequent downstream triggering of tau sticky protein formation in the locus coeruleus that the neuroprotective effects of inhaled lithium are completely overwhelmed. On the other hand, inflammation and oxidative stress in the brain's blood vessels are mostly *not* associated with an increased risk for PD (Table 2, Chapter 1) and should, therefore, not trigger the formation of alpha-synuclein sticky proteins in the olfactory bulb and myenteric plexus. In fact, there are significantly fewer numbers of mini-strokes in PD brains than in the brains of age-matched healthy people, further illustrating that blood vessel pathology—including that caused by smoking cigarettes—is unlikely to be a risk for PD.[78] Therefore, smoking-induced inflammation and oxidative stress in blood vessels occur in a location mostly irrelevant to PD and, thus, would not counteract the neuroprotective effects of inhaled lithium from smoking resulting in a greatly reduced risk of PD in smokers. If all of this is true, then lithium therapy in AD and PD would provide all of lithium's neuroprotective benefits without all of the vascular toxicities and carcinogen exposure from smoking cigarettes.

It is pretty ironic that the most dangerous consumer product available behind the counter at most gas stations may actually be teaching us of a highly effective treatment for the world's two most common neurodegenerative diseases affecting over 45 million people: AD and PD.

If this theory is true, then there should be extensive evidence in both animal studies and in humans who take lithium for bipolar disorder that lithium has great promise for preventing and slowing AD and PD progression. Indeed, this extensive evidence exists and is impressive.

Lithium's History

One of the main reasons that lithium has amassed such an impressive record is that lithium has been around for a very long time and, as such, is the oldest medicine in existence.

Although lithium was not discovered as an element on earth until 1817 and not used as a medicine until the mid-1800s for treating gout, kidney stones, depression, and general nervousness, lithium is much older than 200 years old.[79] The element lithium is one of the first three elements created along with hydrogen and helium over 13 billion years ago during the Big Bang that created the universe. Lithium sits as the third element in the Periodic Table of Elements and is part of the earth and most living and non-living matter on earth. In fact, there are low concentrations of lithium circulating in the bloodstream of humans just like the elements of sodium, potassium, and calcium.[80] Because lithium is an all-natural earth element, this has given researchers the ability to look for natural associations between lithium exposure in the environment and the likelihood for developing various diseases including AD and PD. This type of research is called epidemiology, which can provide important clues as to both causes of and treatments for disease.

For example, it was observations made by epidemiologists that smoking was associated with much higher rates of lung cancer, emphysema, and heart disease that eventually led to the conclusion that smoking actually causes these diseases. We reviewed previously that in some of these same studies, it was observed that smokers also have a 77% reduced rate of developing PD and that the tobacco leaf has very high levels of lithium, which bolstered the theory that lithium may prevent PD and slow PD symptom progression.[81]

Informed observations have led to some of medicine's greatest discoveries, including penicillin as an antibiotic, aspirin as the first medicine to prevent heart attacks, and the vaccine that eradicated smallpox from the world.[82] All of these momentous discoveries that have prevented millions of deaths and untold suffering had their inception when a curious scientist or doctor took notice of an unexpected observation. The take-home message is this: don't discount the power of observation.

Another historical example of the power of observation is the accidental discovery of lithium as an effective treatment for the condition called bipolar disorder.[83]

The Australian psychiatrist John Cade had a hypothesis that mania, a state of irrational euphoria and grandiosity that patients with bipolar disorder experience, was caused by excessive amounts of uric acid in the bloodstream. To test his theory, Cade sought to inject uric acid into guinea pigs to observe if they became manic. In order to make uric acid soluble in water and amenable to injection through a needle, Cade used lithium as a salt carrier for the uric acid. When Cade injected lithium urate into the guinea pigs, to his surprise they all became very calm, which was the exact opposite of what Cade hypothesized would happen. Although Cade must have been disappointed that his theory was incorrect, he quickly pivoted his thinking and wondered if lithium might actually be an effective treatment for mania. When he observed the same calming effect in the guinea pigs after injecting them with another lithium salt, lithium carbonate, Cade was convinced that it was time to try lithium treatment in his manic patients and observe the effects.

In his initial clinical trial, Cade treated 10 manic patients with lithium and, to his delight, observed all 10 to have a near full resolution of their symptoms. He published his findings in 1949; however, the world was slow to believe in Cade's observations. In fact, despite many other subsequent independent reports published in the 1950s confirming Cade's findings, two prominent British psychiatrists dismissed these reports as "dangerous nonsense" and recommended that "lithium must be ravaged with fire and sword."[84] Despite these setbacks, the benefits of lithium in the treatment and prevention of mania were subsequently confirmed in several human clinical trials leading to its approval to treat mania in 49 countries in the 1960s. The United States was far behind other countries and finally approved lithium in 1970, becoming the fiftieth country to do so.

Thus, it took 21 years from Cade's first published observations of lithium's benefits in treating mania before it was FDA-approved in the US. This may seem like a very long period of time for the world to accept a treatment that to this day is still considered to be the most effective treatment for bipolar disorder.[85] Although observations alone are insufficient to guide medical practice, the story of the discovery of lithium as a treatment for bipolar disorder again teaches us that promising observations of novel treatments for serious medical conditions should not be dismissed. Promising observations deserve to be investigated.

Even though lithium proved to be highly effective for treating mania and bipolar disorder, its mechanism of action in the brain remained a mystery. In the late 1990s, researchers embarked on a series of experiments to try to determine why lithium was so effective for treating bipolar disorder. They thought that if they could identify the specific targets in brain cells responsible for lithium's effectiveness, perhaps this knowledge could lead to the development of other effective treatments for bipolar disorder. In yet another example of serendipity, what the researchers accidentally discovered from these experiments was of potentially far greater benefit to public health than their original intentions.[86]

Lithium's Multitude of Neuroprotective Actions

Almost all of the actions that lithium was discovered to have were also known to be neuroprotective actions. That is, lithium could protect brain cells from a variety of insults. Among the insults from which lithium could protect were those stemming from the Brain's Bermuda Triangle: sticky proteins, inflammation, and oxidative stress (Figure 1, Chapter 1). With scientists excited about the potential for lithium to prevent and treat the two most common neurodegenerative disorders, AD and PD, many publications appeared in the scientific literature in the 2000s further exploring this promising new use of lithium.

I will not delve into the details of all of lithium's actions but will list them here simply to show how diverse they are. Lithium was shown to increase the expression of neuroprotective proteins Bcl-2 and BDNF in the brain; suppress microglia activation; reduce inflammation; inhibit oxidative stress by improving mitochondrial health, reproduction, and function; inhibit the enzymes GSK-3B and inositol monophosphatase and stimulate the enzyme called Akt inside brain cells, resulting in neuroprotection through several different pathways including enhancing lysosomal function and decreasing sticky phosphorylation of tau.[87] As reviewed in Chapter 1, a therapy will need to effectively target all three of the destructive processes of the Brain's Bermuda Triangle to maximize its potential to prevent and slow AD and PD. Lithium checks all three boxes since it effectively 1) enhances lysosomal function and decreases sticky protein accumulation; 2) suppresses microglial activation and decreases chronic inflammation; and 3) enhances mitochondrial health, reproduction, and function and decreases oxidative stress.

Equally as important as lithium's ability to reduce the Brain's Bermuda Triangle of destruction is its unique ability to gain unfettered access inside brain cells where lysosomes and mitochondria reside. Many drugs have been shown to engage this intracellular machinery when studied in petri dishes in a laboratory. However, how a drug works in the human body is a whole different story. This is because the brain is protected from potentially harmful substances in the bloodstream by the blood-brain barrier (BBB), as reviewed in Chapter 1. The BBB is a formidable barrier. Unless a drug possesses very specific qualities, it will be denied access into the brain and remain banished to the bloodstream. Dozens of molecules that have shown great promise for treating AD or PD in the laboratory have failed when tested in animals and/or humans because they are denied passage across the BBB. Crossing the BBB is just the first hurdle for a drug intended to treat AD or PD. Once inside the brain, a drug also needs to cross brain cells' outer protective wall, called the plasma membrane, in order to access and engage the intracellular machinery necessary to quell the Brain's Bermuda Triangle. Fortunately, lithium is highly effective at crossing *both* the BBB and brain cells' plasma membranes to gain easy access to intracellular machinery like lysosomes and mitochondria.

How does lithium achieve this easy access? It does so by hitching a ride through the multitude of channels located on these barriers that are primarily used for transporting sodium, which is a critically important brain element necessary for almost all brain activities.[88] Channels are specialized bridges that only allow passage of specific items. Thus, sodium channels allow passage of sodium across the BBB and brain cells' plasma membranes. Because lithium and sodium have a similar size and charge, lithium readily travels with sodium across sodium channels. Not only does lithium gain easy access to the interior of brain cells, but it has been clear ever since Cade's experiments in 1949 that lithium, evident in its efficacy for treating bipolar disorder, induces meaningful clinical effects once inside brain cells. Besides the brain, sodium channels are ubiquitous throughout the body, allowing lithium easy access inside virtually all cells. Thus, lithium could offer benefits to other organs besides the brain. Interestingly, lithium use as well as smoking is also associated with *reduced* rates of a malignant skin cancer called melanoma and an inflammatory bowel disease called ulcerative colitis.[89] These observations suggest that lithium therapy may have a role in the prevention and treatment of these extra-brain conditions, which would not be possible without lithium's ability to gain easy access inside virtually all cells in the body.

Lithium is Effective in AD and PD Animal Models

Because of lithium's breadth of neuroprotective actions, lithium has been tested in several animal models of AD and PD. The results have been remarkable.

Animal models of AD and PD come in two broad categories: toxin-induced and genetic models. With the toxin-induced models, a toxin that is known to damage brain cells in a manner similar to what occurs in actual AD and PD patients is injected into a group of animals, typically mice or rats, and a neuroprotective compound is also administered either before or soon after the toxin is injected. Another group of animals is injected only with the toxin to serve as a control group. The animals are then studied for a few weeks to see if there are any intergroup differences in the animals' symptoms. Finally, the animals are sacrificed to determine if there are any intergroup differences in the degree of brain damage. In the genetic animal models of AD and PD, the same research design is used; however, instead of using a toxin, scientists will alter the genetic code of a group of animals so that they eventually develop many or all of the features of AD or PD. Typically, these genetic alterations have been discovered from patients with AD or PD who have a large number of family members with AD or PD. These inherited forms of AD or PD make up less than 7% of all cases of AD or PD, but they provide an opportunity for scientists to use these discovered genetic alterations and develop genetic animal models for research with the ultimate goal of discovering new treatments.

In both toxin-induced and genetic models of AD and PD, lithium has proven to be highly effective in preventing both symptoms and brain damage. In AD genetic mouse models, lithium treatment led to reduced levels of sticky proteins, reduced brain cell damage, and improved memory abilities.[90] In one of these studies, a lithium dose of only 0.3 mg a day (as a converted human dose) was shown to provide significant benefits to memory and to fully protect brain cells from dying.[91] As with any medication, finding the correct dosage is critically important not only to maximize its effectiveness but also to minimize its side effects. Lithium is no exception. As you will see in Chapter 4, the use of too high of a lithium dose has doomed several previous human clinical trials due to very high rates of side effects in the participating patients. If lithium was found to be effective in AD or PD patients at very low dosages, that would be a huge benefit to patients not only because there would be very little chance for side effects but also because low doses of lithium are available over the counter (OTC) as an inexpensive dietary supplement, which will be reviewed in Chapter 6.

Lithium treatment has also shown remarkable benefits in PD animal models just as it has in AD animal models. As reviewed in Chapter 1, exposure to environmental toxins such as pesticides increases the risk of developing PD. Injection of these pesticides into mice can cause brain damage and symptoms very similar to what is seen in PD patients. These toxin-induced PD animal models have been extensively studied. As expected, lithium has proven to be effective for improving symptoms and reducing brain damage in virtually all of these toxin-induced PD animal models.[92] In addition, lithium has also been effective for improving symptoms and reducing brain damage in several genetic PD animal models.[93]

Although the results from these AD and PD animal studies are very promising, positive results from animal studies are far from a guarantee that similar results will occur in humans. However, if there were any existing human data supporting lithium's ability to prevent and/or slow AD and PD, that would greatly bolster the impact of the promising animal data. Well, guess what? There is a great deal of supporting human evidence. Let's dive into it.

CHAPTER 3

THE HUMAN EVIDENCE

YEARS AGO, A PD PATIENT of mine brought me an article to read about a new treatment that had cured rats of their Parkinson's symptoms and wondered when it would be available for humans with PD to use. I explained to him that it takes many years for promising drugs to work their way into human clinical trials and that the few that had made it that far in the past had all failed when tested in humans. Most of my patients develop a look of disappointment at this point. But this patient developed a smirk and retorted, "This is the first time in my life that I wish I was a rat."

Yes, if only AD and PD patients were rats, they all would have been cured years ago. As with most things in life, we are required to take the good with the bad. Humans have greatly benefited from our advanced cognitive abilities stemming from our expanded brain mass and complexity; however, we also have to contend with diseases like AD and PD that have proven to be very resistant to treatments that often work remarkably well in animal models of AD and PD. So where does that leave us?

How can we get a better sense of whether an effective treatment in animal models of AD or PD will also be effective in humans with AD or PD? Fortunately, with lithium there is already ample human evidence.

Lithium in Drinking Water

Because lithium is a natural earth element found in most living and much non-living matter, this gives researchers the opportunity to look for associations between environmental lithium exposure and disease incidence. Also, because lithium has been FDA-approved for treating bipolar disorder since 1970, researchers can also examine for associations between use of prescription lithium and disease incidence. These are qualities of lithium that make it completely unique compared to the typical drugs that pharmaceutical companies synthesize, patent, and test in animals and then humans. We already reviewed the highly promising animal data on lithium. But since our goal is to treat humans with AD or PD, not rodents, human data are far more important. Let's start with reviewing associations between human behaviors and exposure to very small amounts of lithium in the environment.

A major source of environmental lithium exposure is drinking water.[94] Rain mobilizes lithium from the soil and rock and carries it into municipal water supplies. Lithium concentrations in drinking water vary greatly among municipalities and world regions with some having no detectable lithium and some having levels as high as 5 mg per liter of water, which translates into about 10 mg/day of lithium intake just from drinking water.[95] Because lithium has a calming effect, as initially observed by

John Cade in his guinea pigs, and is a highly effective mood stabilizer for treating bipolar disorder, some of the earliest environmental studies examined associations between lithium concentrations in drinking water and rates of suicide and violent crime among various municipalities. The theory was that suicide and violent crime would be lower in municipalities with the highest levels of lithium in their drinking water due to the calming and mood-stabilizing effects of lithium. This is exactly what several independent studies conducted in different countries have found[96] with only one exception.[97] One study even found a decreased rate of death from any cause in municipalities with higher lithium levels in drinking water.[98] Considering that the number one cause of death in both men and women is heart disease, it's also interesting that way back in 1969 higher lithium levels in drinking water were associated with lower risks of dying from heart disease.[99]

If you were paying attention in Chapter 1, you are hopefully seeing a connection between lithium's association with cardiovascular benefits and its potential to prevent and slow AD. In Chapter 1, we saw that the same risk factors for heart disease (i.e., high blood pressure, diabetes, high cholesterol, and smoking) were all prominent risk factors for developing AD. Now we see that higher intake of environmental lithium in drinking water is associated with a decreased risk of dying from heart disease. Therefore, it would make sense based on all of this background information that higher environmental lithium intake could also be associated with a lower risk for AD. But do such data exist?

In fact, they do. A study in Denmark examined associations between drinking water lithium levels and rates of AD across municipalities over a 19-year period from 1995 to 2013. This study found a significant 22% reduced rate of AD in municipalities with the highest drinking water lithium levels.[100] Although these results fit in with the theory that small amounts of daily lithium intake can prevent AD, in order for study results to be considered reliable they need to be replicated in an independent second study to ensure that the original study results were not a fluke. Surprisingly, the Denmark study results were replicated in a study in Texas the very next year.[101] This study examined associations between drinking water lithium levels, AD mortality, obesity, and diabetes across 234 Texas counties. The results were shocking. Not only did this study replicate the results of the Denmark study by finding that high drinking water lithium levels were associated with significantly reduced rates of AD mortality, but it also found high drinking water lithium levels to be associated with significantly lower rates of obesity and diabetes. Not surprisingly, the study also found obesity and diabetes to be associated with higher rates of AD.

In summary, several studies have now found associations between high drinking water lithium levels and improved health outcomes, including decreased rates of AD, AD mortality, suicide, violent crime, diabetes, obesity, heart disease mortality, and all-cause mortality.

Before you jump up and conclude that it's time to start taking lithium, you should understand that these studies show only associations or correlations between lithium intake and these positive health outcomes. It would be incorrect to draw the conclusion that, based on these studies' findings, daily lithium intake from drinking water is what *caused* these positive health outcomes. In other words, correlation does not equal causation. Let me give you an example that is frequently cited to illustrate this point.

Did you know that eating ice cream is associated with a five-fold increased risk of drowning? Why do you think this is? The first explanation that likely comes to mind is that there is something about eating ice cream that makes it difficult to safely swim. Perhaps eating ice cream lowers your core body temperature or makes it more likely to get abdominal cramps and, therefore, causes a person to drown if they try to swim soon after eating ice cream. The assumption is that eating ice cream somehow *causes* a person to drown. It is natural for the human mind to make such causation conclusions when faced with these types of correlation data. The truth in this example is that ice cream has nothing to do with why people are drowning. There's a completely different, hidden variable that accounts for the increased risk of drowning that is also *correlated* with eating ice cream. And what is that variable? It's hot weather! People eat much more ice cream when it's hot outside than when it's cold. And most drownings occur in the summer when it's hot and people go swimming. So it's the hot weather during summer and not eating ice cream that is the relevant factor accounting for the increased drownings. The point is that correlation does not equal causation, and we must be careful not to jump to conclusions too quickly.

So although it is tempting to conclude that daily intake of small amounts of lithium will prevent AD and heart disease based on the above drinking water studies, we need much more data. What kind of data do we need? It would first be valuable to see if people taking prescription lithium for bipolar disorder have lower rates of AD, PD, or vascular disease, which would help to substantiate the above drinking water study findings. Then it would be most important to see if there were any clinical trial data, especially from "randomized controlled trials" (RCTs), showing that AD or PD patients' symptoms improved when prescribed lithium.

The RCT is the "gold standard," top-of-the-line level of evidence needed in order to prove whether a treatment is effective for treating a disease. Because results from RCTs are so convincing, these are the results the FDA relies upon to approve a medication for use in the US population. That's how important RCTs are to patient care.

The design of an RCT is quite simple: a group of patients are randomly assigned either to treatment with an active drug or an identically appearing inactive drug (called a placebo) in a double-blind manner and followed for a period of time to determine if the patients assigned to the active drug experience a "statistically significant" improvement in their symptoms compared to those assigned to a placebo. Double-blind means that neither the patients nor the members of the research study team know to which treatment each subject has been assigned until the study is completed and the statistician has evaluated the data. Although the double-blind feature of an RCT is important, the majority of the rigor derived from an RCT stems from patient randomization. When a large enough group of patients is randomly assigned to either an active treatment or a placebo, like flipping a coin, both known and unknown variables will be equivalently allocated between the groups. As a result of patient randomization in a large enough sample of patients, differences in patient outcomes can confidently be interpreted as being caused by the treatment and not by some other variable. In other words, the design of the RCT prevents us from making erroneous conclusions—such as the idea that eating ice cream causes people to drown. When it comes to proving that a therapy is effective, there's no level of evidence more rigorous or convincing than positive results from a well-designed RCT.

But this doesn't mean that observational, correlative data should be ignored. It just means we need to be careful not to jump to conclusions too early. Sometimes observational studies prove to be highly valuable to the population, like the initial studies associating smoking with an increased risk of dying from lung cancer, emphysema, and heart disease. Sometimes observational studies lead us completely astray, like the initial studies associating hormone replacement therapy with greatly reduced risks of heart disease, cancer, and dementia in older postmenopausal women—only to have a large, well-designed RCT show the exact opposite results![102] Observational studies raise interesting possibilities for discoveries. But until these observations are formally assessed with RCTs, they remain just possibilities.

Let's take the lithium story to the next level. If tiny amounts of daily lithium intake from drinking water could prevent AD, then higher doses of lithium given as a daily prescription medication to bipolar patients should do the same and perhaps to an even greater extent.

Prescription Lithium Use

Because lithium is mainly prescribed to patients with bipolar disorder who are known to be at increased risk for developing

AD compared to people without bipolar disorder, these factors need to be accounted for when interpreting the results from prescription lithium observational studies.[103] For example, if a study showed that bipolar disorder patients taking lithium had similar rates of AD as people without bipolar disorder not taking lithium, it would be hard to draw any meaningful conclusions because there would be too many variables at play. Thus, most studies have focused just on bipolar disorder patients and have compared disease incidence among patients taking different treatments for their bipolar disorder.

One of the first such studies was performed in Brazil and found a significantly reduced rate of AD among 66 bipolar disease patients receiving continuous lithium treatment for almost six years versus a similar group of 48 bipolar disease patients treated with other psychiatric drugs who had either never received lithium or had received lithium in the past but had stopped it for about five years.[104] These study results were subsequently confirmed in several other studies, one of which showed as much as a 62% reduced risk of dementia in bipolar patients receiving lithium compared to those not receiving lithium.[105] A 2022 study showed a whopping 70% reduced risk of AD in patients receiving lithium for more than five years compared to patients not receiving lithium.[106] In this particular study, there were significantly more smokers and people with bipolar disorder, depression, hypertension, diabetes, and stroke in the lithium-treated group than the comparison group, which are all factors associated with an *increased*, not decreased, risk for AD.[107] Despite all of these factors, there was still a 70% reduced risk of AD in patients treated with lithium for more than five years.

A 70% AD risk reduction is very large and over three times as much as the 22% AD risk reduction observed in municipalities with high drinking water lithium levels.[108] Perhaps these differences are due to differences in the design of these studies, or perhaps they are due to the fact that bipolar disorder patients receive a much higher daily elemental lithium dosage (about 160–400 mg/day) than those living in the municipalities with high drinking water lithium levels that had a decreased risk of AD (about 0.06 mg/day).[109] We will talk about lithium dosing in much greater detail in Chapter 6. The take-home message is that both small and larger doses of daily lithium are associated with a reduced risk of developing AD, as much as a 70% reduced risk.

If daily lithium intake can decrease the risk of AD, and the main risks for AD are vascular risk factors that lead to blood vessel inflammation, oxidative stress, and small vessel strokes (as reviewed in Chapter 1), it is not surprising that prescription lithium use is also associated with a greatly reduced risk of stroke (as high as an 80% reduced risk) and reduced build-up of the fatty plaques in arteries that lead to stroke.[110] There even is "gold-standard" evidence from an RCT supporting lithium as a potential treatment for patients with a recent stroke to improve their neurological recovery.[111] The association of lithium therapy with significantly improved vascular health in humans may partially explain why lithium is also associated with a significantly reduced risk of developing AD. The pieces of the puzzle are coming together.

What about PD? As reviewed in Chapter 1, both AD and PD are caused by the Brain's Bermuda Triangle of accumulating sticky proteins, inflammation, and oxidative stress. Because lithium successfully targets all three processes as reviewed in Chapter 2, is there evidence that use of prescription lithium is associated with a reduced risk of PD just like AD? Actually, there is not. In fact, one study showed that older patients taking prescription lithium actually have a significantly higher rate of being diagnosed with PD or being prescribed PD medications compared to patients taking antidepressant medications.[112] How could this be if lithium is supposed to prevent PD? The answer may lie in Paracelsus's quote from the sixteenth century: "The dose makes the poison."

Lithium embodies this principle perfectly. As effective as lithium is for treating bipolar disorder, too high of a dosage can cause dangerous and even lethal side effects. This is why lithium blood levels need to be monitored in patients receiving lithium in order to make sure that they are taking the correct dosage. However, even at the correct dosage for bipolar disorder, it is important to note that 25–50% of patients develop lithium-induced hand tremors, which is shaking of the hands.[113] Although lithium-induced hand tremors are of a different quality than PD hand tremors, the two types of tremors are often confused with each other by doctors, which could easily account for why older patients receiving lithium may be misdiagnosed as having PD.[114] Interestingly, when comparing older patients taking lithium to older patients taking a medication called valproic acid, which also frequently causes hand tremors, lithium use is no longer associated with a higher rate of PD diagnosis or greater use of PD medications.[115] These findings suggest that drug-induced hand tremors, whether from lithium or valproic acid, can be misdiagnosed as PD.

It is also important to note that the occurrence of lithium-induced hand tremors is dose dependent. A fairly high dosage of elemental lithium (about 160–400 mg/day) is required to effectively treat bipolar disorder and can also cause lithium-induced hand tremors. However, studies have shown that when much lower dosages of prescription lithium (about half of the bipolar disorder dosage) are given to elderly patients, there is no increase in hand tremors.[116] The public databases that have been examined for associations between lithium use and rates of AD or PD consist almost completely of bipolar disorder or depression patients receiving higher dosages of lithium. Because about 25–50% of these patients would be expected to have lithium-induced hand tremors, many of these tremulous patients may be misdiagnosed as having PD, but virtually none will be misdiagnosed as having AD since AD patients do not have hand tremors. It would not take many patients with lithium-induced tremors to be misdiagnosed and recorded as having PD in these databases to completely negate the detection of lithium-induced protection against developing PD. However, such PD misdiagnoses would not affect the detection of lithium-induced protection against AD, which is exactly what these databases have shown.[117]

In short, the tremor side effect of lithium renders these public databases fairly useless for examining if lithium can prevent PD. However, as reviewed in Chapter 1, the very small daily dosages of lithium inhaled from smoking a pack of cigarettes (about 0.3 mg/day) would be far too low of a dose to cause tremors and, therefore, would not mask lithium-induced neuroprotective effects that may account for the 77% reduced risk of PD observed in smokers.[118] Although a small daily dosage of lithium from drinking water has been associated with lower rates of AD, unfortunately, no such similar studies have been performed to date examining for rates of PD in municipalities with high versus low lithium levels in drinking water.[119] Such a study would be highly valuable to the field and hopefully will be performed in the near future.

In addition to inhaled lithium from smoking being associated with a decreased risk for PD, there is another tangential line of human evidence supporting this association. Strangely enough, it has to do with the skin cancer melanoma.

Lithium and Melanoma

Melanoma is a malignant skin cancer that is found in PD patients at three times the rate as in non-PD patients of the same age.[120] This association between melanoma and PD has been known for almost 20 years without a reasonable explanation. Furthermore, having a personal or a family history of melanoma—but not of other cancers like colorectal, lung, prostate, or breast cancer— is associated with a significant increased risk for PD.[121] These observations suggest that PD and melanoma share common risks or causative disease pathways that, if revealed, could help to discover new therapeutic targets and treatments for both conditions. As further support, studies show that male smokers have a significant 37–47% decreased risk of developing melanoma with as much as a 68% reduced melanoma risk associated with smoking more than 15 cigarettes per day.[122]

Smoking can lead to a decreased risk of cancer?! Sounds crazy, but these are the data. At this point, I hope that you are starting to see some connections. As reviewed in Chapter 1, smoking is also associated with a 77% reduced risk of PD, which may be due to the very high lithium levels found in the tobacco leaf that would be inhaled and absorbed through the lungs when smoking.[123] Because smoking is associated with reduced risks of both PD and melanoma, could it be that lithium positively engages a common disease pathway thus leading to reduced rates of both diseases?

It turns out that there is a biological pathway implicated in both PD and melanoma. It's called the beta-catenin pathway.[124] Beta-catenin is a protein that, when concentrated in a cell, can increase the expression of many different genes. One of the genes under the control of beta-catenin is called Nurr1 (nuclear receptor-related 1 protein).[125] Nurr1 is a protein that is particularly important for maintaining the health and survival of dopamine-producing brain cells, which are the exact brain cells that progressively die in PD and lead to the symptoms of tremor, stiffness, and slowness of movement upon which a PD diagnosis is made.[126] Nurr1 levels are significantly reduced by over 60% in PD patients' dopamine brain cells and circulating white blood cells compared to people of similar age without PD.[127] Also, brain cell Nurr1 expression progressively decreases by 46% with normal human aging, which is the major risk factor for PD and has been implicated in the most common inherited causes of PD.[128] These findings suggest that therapies that can increase Nurr1 levels may be capable of preventing and slowing PD. As it turns out, lithium has been shown to increase Nurr1 levels by about 180% as well as protect cells in a model of PD.[129] You will see in Chapter 5 that lithium therapy in patients with PD was recently shown to increase Nurr1 levels by as much as 679%, which is good news since Nurr1 is known to help protect brain cells.

Decreased beta-catenin is also implicated in melanoma occurrence, and lithium can inhibit melanoma proliferation.[130] Finally, a human study showed that use of prescription lithium was associated with a significantly reduced incidence of melanoma as well as reduced melanoma-associated mortality.[131]

Although PD is associated with higher rates of melanoma, surprisingly, PD is also associated with significantly lower rates of several non-skin cancers—including colorectal, hematologic, prostate, and lung cancers—and a lower risk of dying from cancer.[132] These disparities in cancer incidences in PD patients may also be related to beta-catenin. For example, reduced beta-catenin activity has been implicated in melanoma occurrence while increased beta-catenin activity has been implicated in the occurrences of many other cancers, especially colorectal cancer.[133] In this way, melanoma is unique among cancers. Thus, reduced beta-catenin activity in PD may partially explain both the associated increased incidence of melanoma and decreased incidences of other cancers. Because lithium increases beta-catenin activity, there would be a theoretical risk for lithium to increase the incidence of non-melanoma cancers.[134] However, use of prescription lithium has not been associated with increased incidences of any cancers, and one study even showed a decreased incidence of cancer associated with use of lithium.[135]

In summary, lithium use *in humans*—whether from drinking water with high lithium content, inhaling lithium from smoking cigarettes, or taking prescription lithium medication—is associated with as much as a 70% reduced risk of developing AD, a

77% reduced risk of PD, and as much as a 68% reduced risk of melanoma, which is relevant because melanoma and PD share a common biological pathway (i.e., the beta-catenin pathway) known to be positively engaged by lithium.

Despite all of this very promising human evidence, the question that remains to be answered is, can lithium therapy slow the progression of AD and PD in clinical trials? If the answer to this question is yes and if lithium therapy can slow AD and PD progression by 70–77%, lithium would truly be a game-changing therapy. Patients with AD and PD would have profoundly improved futures with far less disability and, if a large percentage of patients took lithium, governments would save billions of dollars every year on the care of AD and PD patients. Several small clinical trials have already been performed to try to answer these questions. Let's review their results now.

Clinical Trials with Lithium: The Highest Level of Evidence

Once you get to the point where it's time to test a drug in a controlled clinical trial, one of the most important questions that needs to be answered is this: what is the correct dosage to study? There is no medication that is effective at any dosage. All medications have an optimal dosage or dosage range where benefits outweigh side effects. If you pick the wrong dosage to study in a clinical trial, the study will fail either because the dosage is too low to provide benefit or too high for patients to tolerate. In either case, the trial will fail to answer the fundamental question of whether or not the medication is effective for the condition being studied.

Unfortunately, most of the clinical trials using lithium for neurodegenerative diseases including AD and PD have used too high of a dosage resulting in too many patients developing intolerable side effects and dropping out of the trials. These early studies made the mistake of assuming that the lithium dosage known to be effective for bipolar disorder, a dosage producing a blood serum lithium level of 0.6–1.2 mmol/L, would also be the optimal dosage to study in AD and PD. This proved to be completely incorrect.

One of the first controlled trials using lithium in a neurodegenerative disease was performed at Duke Medical Center in 1982 among six PD patients, which was already discussed in detail at the beginning of Chapter 2.[136] Briefly, this study initially showed promising results when PD patients received a lithium dosage producing a serum lithium level of 0.8 mmol/L. However, all five patients who continued lithium therapy at this dosage eventually developed severe side effects called dyskinesias, and three of the five needed to stop lithium treatment.[137] After this study, very little research was performed using lithium in PD patients until 2014 when my PD patient Ted (discussed earlier) told me that his motor fluctuations almost fully resolved after his psychiatrist prescribed him a low dosage of lithium for his concomitant bipolar disorder. Ted's serum lithium level at that time was only 0.4 mmol/L. After seeing that Ted experienced no side effects or dyskinesias from this low dosage of lithium for over six months, I theorized that perhaps low-dose lithium therapy could provide benefits to PD patients with motor fluctuations without the side effects previously found by the Duke group when using about twice the lithium dose. I have now prescribed a similar low dose of lithium (target serum level being 0.4–0.5 mmol/L) to 20 other PD patients and have found it to be well tolerated in patients without dementia and, anecdotally, to be associated with remarkable improvements in PD motor fluctuations.[138] This discovery was purely accidental. If Ted's psychiatrist had not prescribed him lithium in 2014, I doubt I would have ever become interested in lithium and certainly would never have written this book.

It turns out a very similar story has played out in AD with too high of a lithium dosage being used in the initial AD clinical trials. The first clinical trial enrolled 22 AD patients with an average age of 81 years old who had more advanced cognitive impairment.[139] The lithium dosage was adjusted until patients achieved an average serum lithium level of 0.4 mmol/L; however, the range among the patients was very wide, spanning from 0.19–0.99 mmol/L. Fourteen of the 22 enrolled patients did not complete the trial primarily due to side effects and had serum lithium levels as high as 0.99 mmol/L. In contrast, the eight patients who completed the 39-week trial had much tighter control of their serum lithium levels, all falling between 0.37–0.49mmol/L and tended to be younger and less cognitively impaired. However, there was no apparent cognitive benefit from lithium therapy for these eight patients that completed the trial compared to a separate control group. Considering how small this study was and that 64% of enrolled patients withdrew, no conclusions could be drawn regarding lithium's benefit in treating AD. However, it did appear that younger, less cognitively impaired AD patients tolerated lower dosages of lithium fairly well.

The next clinical trial enrolled AD patients with an average age of 68 years old with less cognitive impairment than the previous trial.[140] Seventy-four AD patients were randomly assigned to either lithium or a placebo for 10 weeks. Patients receiving lithium had an average serum lithium level of 0.68 mmol/L at week 10. This study did not find any differences between the lithium and placebo groups for a variety of blood and cerebrospinal fluid markers of AD disease activity (aka biomarkers), nor for cognitive abilities in the patients. There were more side effects in the lithium group but not a greater number of patient withdrawals. Although this second study did not have such a large patient drop-out rate like the first study (perhaps because patients were younger with less severe cognitive impairment compared to the first study), it was only 10 weeks in duration. This is much too short of a period of time to expect to see changes in either biomarkers or cognition in AD patients. Thus, this study design also failed to answer the question of whether lithium has benefit for treating AD.

The next two AD trials, both of which were conducted in Brazil, sought to correct the trial design flaws of the first two studies by using much longer lithium treatment periods and much lower lithium dosages to hopefully reduce patient side effects and withdrawals.

The first Brazilian study enrolled patients with a pre-AD condition called amnestic mild cognitive impairment (aMCI), which is a condition that primarily involves impairment in short-term memory abilities. About 30–50% of aMCI patients go on to develop AD within three years, making aMCI one of the strongest predictors of future AD.[141] These researchers theorized that if lithium could prevent AD, then aMCI would be the perfect group to study. Introducing a neuroprotective treatment in the earliest stages of the AD process would enable protection of the greatest number of brain cells and, therefore, the greatest chance to demonstrate cognitive benefits and prevent conversion from aMCI to AD. As Benjamin Franklin stated in 1736, "An ounce of prevention is worth a pound of cure." In other words, it is preferable and easier to prevent a disease from occurring in the first place than to wait for it to take hold and then try to cure it.

In addition to examining for any benefits to cognition, this Brazilian clinical trial also examined for any benefits lithium may have to AD biomarkers in the cerebrospinal fluid (CSF) of patients. The brain and spinal cord are bathed in CSF, which acts as a watery cushion to support and protect the brain. Disease processes such as accumulating sticky proteins inside brain cells can leach out of the cells and into the CSF and the bloodstream. A sample of CSF can be easily obtained by inserting a thin needle in between two of the lower bones of the spine and into the spinal canal, a procedure called a spinal tap or lumbar puncture. Because these sticky protein biomarkers are known to reflect the disease process in the brain, as reviewed in Chapter 1, a therapy that could positively affect these biomarkers would imply that the therapy could slow down the disease process and improve patients' long-term prognoses. In our quest to discover a "disease-modifying therapy" for AD and PD, the use of biomarkers in clinical trials is of paramount importance. We will take a much deeper dive into the use of biomarkers in AD and PD clinical trials in Chapter 5.

Now, let's review the design and exciting results of this first Brazilian RCT performed by Forlenza et al. at the University of Sao Paulo.[142] This study enrolled 45 patients with aMCI and randomly assigned them, in a double-blind fashion, to therapy with either lithium (23 patients) or placebo (22 patients) for 12 months. "Double-blind" means that both the researchers and the patients did not know which treatment patients were receiving, and the lithium and placebo pills appeared identical. For the patients receiving lithium, the target serum lithium range was 0.25–0.5 mmol/L, which would equate to an elemental lithium dosage of about 80–200 mg/day depending on the individual. A much lower target lithium level was chosen compared to previous studies in order to improve lithium's tolerability and, thus, avoid patients withdrawing from the study. The authors stated that they had evidence showing that this lower serum lithium level engaged an important blood biomarker lithium target: GSK-3B inhibition. Selecting an ideal lithium dosage to study based on the degree of biomarker engagement was also used in a PD clinical trial that will be reviewed in Chapter 5. Forlenza et al. measured many different cognitive tests in the aMCI patients at baseline and after 12 months of treatment, as well as several CSF biomarkers including the particular sticky protein that accumulates inside brain cells and CSF in AD patients: p-tau.[143] Therefore, in AD, CSF p-tau levels are increased.

The results showed that after 12 months of therapy, the patients receiving lithium *did not* show any significant worsening in their cognition as measured by the gold-standard cognitive assessment instrument called the Alzheimer's Disease Assessment Scale-Cognitive Subscale (ADAS-Cog), while the patients receiving placebo *did* show a significant decline on the ADAS-Cog. Specifically, the lithium and placebo groups showed worsening in ADAS-Cog scores over 12 months of 1.6 ($p=0.21$) and 3.2 ($p=0.03$) points, respectively. A *p* value less than 0.05 indicates that there is a "statistically significant difference" between groups of numbers and is the conventional statistical cutoff value for determining a "significant difference." Thus, both groups showed numerical declines in cognition reflected in ADAS-Cog scores, but the lithium group declined *at about half the rate* (1.6 points) as the placebo group (3.2 points). Reflecting this slower rate of decline, 42% fewer patients in the lithium group progressed from aMCI to AD as in the placebo group; however, due to the small number of patients enrolled in this study, this difference between groups did not reach statistical significance (p=0.2). Finally, the lithium group showed *a significant decrease* in CSF p-tau levels compared to *an increase* in p-tau found in the placebo group over the 12-month study (p=0.02). Patients tolerated this low dose of lithium very well, evident in the equivalent rates of side effects in patients taking lithium versus those taking placebo therapy. A two-year follow-up analysis including most of the patients from this study and some additional aMCI patients showed very similar results.[144]

The implications from the results of the Forlenza et al. study are profound. This study showed that in those at greatest risk for developing AD, low-dose lithium therapy slows cognitive decline, likely slows the destructive process of sticky protein accumulation in the brain, and may decrease the likelihood of developing AD by 42%. These are extremely impressive results for the first study of its kind and clearly warrant further research on low-dose lithium therapy in aMCI and AD.

The results from the second study performed in Brazil were in some ways more and some ways less impressive than those from the Forlenza et al. study. This study performed by Nunes et al. was also a randomized, double-blind, placebo-controlled trial (RCT); however, instead of enrolling aMCI patients, this study enrolled 113 patients who had already developed AD.[145] Other unique features of this study were that 1) a "microdose" of lithium was used (0.3 mg of elemental lithium/day compared to the 80–200 mg/day dosage used by Forlenza et al.); 2) treatment lasted for 15 months instead of 12 months; 3) the only cognitive assessment was a simple test called the Mini-Mental State Exam (MMSE) that was assessed every three months; and 4) no biomarkers were assessed. During the study, nine patients in the lithium group and 10 in the placebo group did not provide complete MMSE data and were excluded from the final analyses. This means that about 17% of the patients enrolled into the study were excluded from the final results, which is a high percentage of patients. Because this study's results were so impressive, as you will soon see, I contacted this research group in Brazil and asked them to send us all of their data from this study, including those from the 17% of patients that they excluded, so that our statistician at the University at Buffalo (UB) could repeat the analyses including *all* enrolled patients. I wanted to determine if we could confirm the results that Nunes et al. reported when all enrolled patients were included in the analysis. This research group agreed and sent us their complete data set. Let's review all of these results.

In the original Nunes et al. paper, after only three months of therapy, there was already a statistically significant difference between the two groups, with the lithium group having higher (better) MMSE scores than the placebo group ($p < 0.01$).[146] Even more surprising was that the lithium group showed no decline at all in MMSE scores over 15 months of treatment, while the placebo group showed a steady decline (worsening) in MMSE scores. As a result, the intergroup differences after 12 and 15 months of treatment had grown to achieve even more convincing degrees of statistical significance ($p<0.001$ at both 12 and 15 months). Because of this widening intergroup difference over time, this study's results implied that 0.3 mg/day of lithium was slowing down the progressive worsening of AD symptoms over time. Furthermore, when our UB statistician repeated the analyses on the original data set from this study including *all* enrolled patients, we saw virtually the exact same results (Figure 4). Although this study only used the simple MMSE cognitive measure instead of the more comprehensive, gold-standard ADAS-Cog measure as was used in the Forlenza et al. study, the Nunes et al. results are shocking.

FIGURE 4:
EFFECT OF LITHIUM 0.3MG/DAY ON COGNITION IN ALZHEIMER'S DISEASE
INCLUDING ALL ENROLLED PATIENTS FROM NUNES ET AL. TRIAL

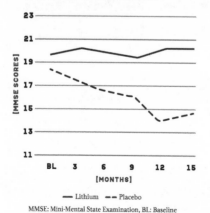

MMSE: Mini-Mental State Examination, BL: Baseline

Figure 4 data courtesy of Hudson Sousa Buck. Statistically significant intergroup differences are observed at 3, 6 and 9 months (p<0.01) and 12 and 15 months (p<0.001).

To put this all into perspective, it was major headline news when the FDA approved the drug aducanumab for treating AD in 2021 despite the fact that most of the clinical trial data showed that aducanumab *did not* slow cognitive decline compared to AD patients taking a placebo. The FDA approved aducanumab based mostly on brain imaging changes that most experts believe do not reflect any benefit to AD patients. On the other hand, the Nunes et al. trial showed that AD patients taking only 0.3 mg of lithium/day had absolutely no decline in cognition for 15 months, while those taking a placebo showed a predictable steady decline, and the difference between the two groups increased over time (Figure 4).[147] If lithium was a patented compound being studied by a major pharmaceutical company and these results were announced, it would be blockbuster news on every news outlet. Unless you lived under a rock, it would be nearly impossible to miss this news. Yet the Nunes et al. and Forlenza et al. trials generated almost no publicity despite their very impressive results. What a shame.

The hope from the observational studies previously reviewed in this chapter was that lithium could slow AD progression by as much as 70%.[148] The combined results from the Forlenza et al. and Nunes et al. RCTs showed that low-dose lithium therapy slowed cognitive decline by about 75% (i.e., the average of the 50% and 100% slowing of cognitive decline found in each study, respectively). If this magnitude of benefit could be replicated in a larger clinical trial along with positive biomarker results, such as reduced CSF p-tau levels, it would represent a game-changing advance in the care of AD. But until such a clinical trial is performed, many will continue to question how such a small daily dosage of lithium (i.e., 0.3 mg) could have this much benefit for a disease as ruthless and complicated as AD. It sounds too good to be true, doesn't it?

When hearing that something sounds "too good to be true," our knee-jerk reaction is to believe that it must be false. But we're not talking about an anecdotal testimonial from a single AD patient who made a YouTube video stating that they had great benefit from some treatment. We're talking about results from two RCTs, which represent the gold-standard, top-of-the-line level of evidence. The Nunes et al. and the Forlenza et al. RCTs trials had their design flaws, which have been discussed. But let's not allow perfect be the enemy of good. These RCTs are not perfect, but they are certainly good. And in the broad context of all the supportive animal model and human data reviewed in this chapter and in Chapter 2, the results from the Forlenza et al. and Nunes et al. trials are clearly good enough to justify larger RCTs with more rigorous study designs and comprehensive biomarkers to show the world if this simple treatment really is effective for slowing AD progression and improving AD patients' futures. What a gift that would be for the 35 million people in the world living with AD, especially considering that small doses of lithium are safe and readily available over the counter as a dietary supplement. Although such RCTs have yet to be performed in PD, small daily lithium doses could have just as much or even greater benefit for PD patients.[149]

So what's the hold up? It has been nine and 11 years since the Nunes et al. and Forlenza et al. study results were published, respectively. What's taking so long for larger RCTs to be performed?

CHAPTER 4

WHAT'S THE HOLD UP?

IT'S HARD TO KNOW FOR SURE, but the idea that an old medication FDA-approved since 1970 that's also available as an OTC dietary supplement could be effective for preventing and slowing AD and PD likely leads to the frequent conclusion that "it's too good to be true." Understanding human nature, this concept may represent the strongest barrier to the further development of lithium for treating AD and PD.

In order to fully appreciate the tenacity of such a barrier, it will be worthwhile to take a short trip to the days of nautical exploration and colonization in the fifteenth to eighteenth centuries and review the story of a disease called scurvy, the parallels it has to the story of lithium, and the convoluted course before the world finally accepted the treatment for scurvy that had been observed to work over 300 years earlier.

Scurvy was a gruesome and fatal disease that killed over two million sailors in the fifteenth to eighteenth centuries. Over this time period, it is believed that more sailors died of scurvy than war, shipwreck, or other diseases combined.[150] The earliest symptom of scurvy was lethargy so intense that sailors could barely find the energy to even stand up. This was followed by severe joint aches and blood blisters in the legs that progressed into the torso, arms, and face. The gums would become spongy, the breath putrid, and the teeth loose until they all fell out. Old wounds would open, and mucous membranes would easily bleed. Left untreated, scurvy led to death, usually from a sudden internal hemorrhage.

With such a horrific and common disease as scurvy, at least among sailors, one of the strangest things about its history is that people kept stumbling upon cures and then forgetting them. Finding a cure for scurvy would have been highly valuable for the kings and the countries possessing the secret remedy. Healthy sailors meant more time at sea to discover the passage to Asia's riches and an immense advantage during battles at sea. Despite this clear financial motivation from the governments of the day, it took almost 300 years from the first published account of the observation that ingestion of certain plants could cure scurvy before the world finally accepted this treatment as fact, with citrus being the most effective treatment.

The first documented observation of a potential cure for scurvy was from the French explorer Jacques Cartier. In December of 1535, Jacques Cartier wrote that after his ships had become locked in ice in the St. Lawrence River at an Iroquois settlement that is now Quebec City, his crew began developing the gruesome condition of scurvy that spread quickly among the 110 men.[151] By February 1536, eight of his men were dead followed by 15 more the following month with only three members, including Cartier, being unaffected by scurvy. Desperate for a scurvy treatment before all of his crew perished, Cartier learned that over 50 Iroquois natives on land had died of the same condition with symptom onset a bit earlier than his crew. Cartier explains that he encountered an Iroquois native named Domagaia who was afflicted with this condition only 10–12 days earlier but was now "whole and sound." Cartier inquired how Domagaia cured himself. Domagaia told Cartier that he did so by drinking a tea made from the bark and needles of a native tree that likely was the eastern white cedar, spruce, or pine. Domagaia provided some branches from this "tree of life" for Cartier and prepared a tea for his crew. After drinking it two or three times, the crew "recovered health and strength, thanks be to God."[152]

About 30 years after Cartier's report of the "tree of life" cure for scurvy, Dutch sailors discovered that lemons and oranges appeared to cure scurvy. Later in the 1500s and 1600s several other ship captains suggested that certain fruits and vegetables could cure scurvy. In 1734 a physician named Johann Bachstrom came up with the term *antiscorbutic* ("without scurvy") referring to eating fresh fruits and vegetables, thus becoming the first person known to suggest that scurvy might be a deficiency disease.[153]

Nevertheless, despite all of these documented observations of scurvy treatments over a 200-year span from Cartier's first report in 1536 to Bachstrom's writings in 1734, hundreds of thousands of sailors continued to die of scurvy. One of the largest and best-documented losses of lives at sea to scurvy occurred during a circumnavigation voyage under the command of British Captain George Anson in 1740.[154] Of the 1,854 men aboard Anson's fleet, 1,666 died allegedly mostly from scurvy over the four-year voyage.

It is unclear if seventeenth- and eighteenth-century ship captains, like Anson, were unaware of the previous reports by Cartier, Dutch sailors, and Bachstrom about the various effective treatments for scurvy or were aware of these reports but, without an endorsement from the medical experts of the time, casually dismissed these simple treatments as nonsense or "too good to be true." After all, maybe it was just a coincidence that sailors recovered from scurvy after drinking Domagaia's tea or eating oranges or vegetables. Maybe these sailors would have recovered anyway, or maybe it was something else that they ate that was the curative agent. When you're the captain of a ship under your king's command, you didn't want to be instituting unendorsed and possibly risky practices with your crew who were essential to your success.

Imagine that you were captain of a seventeenth-century British ship, and you ordered your men to drink a tea made from some strange plant in order to prevent a condition that they may or may not get, and your entire crew died. Say goodbye to ever being a captain again. In fact, upon returning home, your king may have ordered you to drink the same tea that you gave to your men. It was known for centuries that certain plants, like hemlock, were highly poisonous. The point being, if you are in a position of authority, it behooves you to be risk averse. On the other hand, if you were George Anson returning to England in 1744 with only 188 crew members still alive, you would likely be seeing the whole risk/benefit ratio of administering a scurvy treatment to your crew far differently than four years earlier when you embarked on your journey with a crew of 1,854. As we reviewed in detail in the previous chapter, the way to determine if promising observations are valid is to perform a clinical trial.

And this is exactly what the British naval surgeon James Lind did on May 20, 1747 aboard the HMS Salisbury ship, which is believed to be the very first clinical trial ever performed.[155] The HMS Salisbury had been at sea for about two months when scurvy broke out among the crew. Lind gathered 12 men with scurvy and assigned two men each to six different treatments while keeping everything else in their diets the same. With this trial design, Lind could state that improvements to scurvy symptoms in any group could be attributed to their assigned treatment and not to some other variable. Lind could also compare the magnitude of benefits among the treatments. In this sense, it was a "controlled" clinical trial. The six treatments that Lind administered were daily intake of the following: a quart of cider, 25 drops of elixir of vitriol (sulfuric acid), six spoonfuls of vinegar, a half a pint of seawater, two oranges and one lemon, and a spicy paste with barley water. The results of this trial were definitive: scurvy symptoms improved quickly in the two men who received two oranges and one lemon a day while the other five groups showed no improvements except for some slight improvements in the cider group. After just six days of daily citrus intake, one of these men was fully recovered and back to full ship duty, and the other was almost fully recovered. The results of this clinical trial certainly appeared to be clear cut: citrus cures scurvy. However, this was the very first scurvy clinical trial ever performed and was very small in size. Similar to the current interpretations of the results of the AD trials by Forlenza et al. and Nunes et al. using low-dose lithium, the medical community back then likely questioned if Lind's results could really be trusted.

Based on Lind's 459-page book that he published in 1753

titled *A Treatise of the Scurvy*, it appears that even Lind himself may not have fully trusted the results of his own study. Lind barely even mentioned his clinical trial results, which he quickly summarized on pages 191–196 buried in the middle of the book.[156] Instead of focusing on his study results, which were by far the most valuable part of his book, Lind focused on his own explanation of scurvy: that it was actually a digestive disease caused by blocked sweat glands. To this day James Lind is the person who gets the most credit for establishing that citrus fruit cures scurvy, and yet, he nearly overlooked his own discovery by getting bogged down in obtuse disease theories instead of focusing on a very simple disease cure.[157] Lind believed that scurvy had many different causes and, therefore, necessitated many different types of treatments for it to be effectively cured.[158] As a result, Lind never advocated citrus as a single solution for treating scurvy, despite the dramatic and rapid benefits that citrus intake had on scurvy, which he personally observed during his own clinical trial in 1747.

The belief that such a simple treatment was "too good to be true" may have been just as much of a barrier to the acceptance of citrus as a treatment for scurvy when Lind published his book in 1753 as it is now regarding lithium treatment for AD and PD. Just as Lind believed that scurvy had many different causes and, therefore, needed many different types of treatments, many researchers today propose the same logic for preventing and slowing AD and PD. Albert Einstein wisely stated, "Everything should be made as simple as possible, but not simpler." Could it be that researchers are getting bogged down in obtuse disease theories and overlooking a simple and effective AD and

PD treatment, lithium, that has been available as a prescription medication since 1970 and is readily available as an OTC dietary supplement? In other words, are the mistakes of history repeating themselves again?

It took a large-scale citrus success story in 1794 witnessed by a person of influence, Admiral Alan Gardner, to get the attention of the British Royal Navy. Familiar with the work of Lind and others, Admiral Gardner insisted that lemon juice be supplied to his crew on the HMS Suffolk for the 23-week, nonstop voyage to India even though this intervention went against the prevailing medical opinion of the time. When no serious cases of scurvy occurred on Gardner's voyage, physician Gilbert Blane was then able to use Gardner's observations to convince the British Royal Navy to issue daily lemon juice to British sailors in 1795; this allowed a prolonged British naval blockade at sea without scurvy in the crew, which was a primary factor in Britain's successfully defending itself against a French invasion. Who knows, perhaps France would have colonized England in 1795, making French and not English the world's universal language if it wasn't for some people of influence (Gardner and Blane) believing in the power of observation and insisting on providing lemon juice to the British crew. Based on these successes, lemon- or lime-juice–supplemented rum became standard fare on British ships in the early 1800s, which proved to be highly effective for preventing scurvy in the crew. It wasn't until 1928 that the curative compound in fruits and vegetables for scurvy was identified as vitamin C.

Thus, it took almost 400 years from Cartier's first observation in 1536 of tea made from the "tree of life" being a cure for scurvy before this cure was understood and universally accepted as true medical knowledge. The story of using vitamin C dietary supplementation for treating and preventing scurvy is now history. The story of using lithium dietary supplementation for treating and preventing AD and PD is still being told.

The scurvy success story should be a lesson to patients and to the medical community to resist making snap judgments regarding an observation of a treatment that appears "too good to be true" or "too simple" for a complex disease. When unexpected and promising observations occur, even if they appear too good to be true, they should be pursued and developed. After all, this is how penicillin and the smallpox vaccine were discovered, which stand as perhaps the two most monumental advances in public health.[159] Although lithium dietary supplementation will never be as effective for AD and PD as vitamin C supplementation is for scurvy, it very well may turn out to be an effective treatment for these conditions that could greatly improve public health in our aging population. We just need to perform larger, well-designed, randomized controlled trials (RCTs) to find out how lithium's story ends.

Besides the medical community's inclination to discount simple treatments as being "too good to be true" or "too simple" to ever work, are there any other obstacles to further developing lithium's story for treating AD and PD? There are actually several. The next obstacle we will discuss may be the most consequential, as it is the one that makes funding agencies very hesitant to grant the funds required to perform larger RCTs. It's the misconception that since lithium has failed in some previous clinical trials, it will fail in future clinical trials.

Once a Failure, Always a Failure

Besides the two initial AD clinical trials reviewed in Chapter 3 that failed potentially due to too high of a lithium dosage or too short of a treatment duration being used, there have been several other clinical trials conducted using lithium to treat other neurodegenerative disorders besides AD and PD that have also not fared so well.[160] Unfortunately, there were also major flaws in these studies' designs that contributed to their negative results. Let's review these trials and see if the negative results justify any tempered enthusiasm for lithium's potential for treating AD and PD.

There are several neurodegenerative conditions that have symptoms similar to PD but have some additional symptoms and qualities to merit distinct diagnoses. Just like AD and PD, these other neurodegenerative conditions are also caused by accumulating and spreading sticky proteins, inflammation, and oxidative stress. Two of these conditions are progressive supranuclear palsy (PSP) and corticobasal degeneration (CBD) both of which have similar changes in the brain and, therefore, are often studied together. A clinical trial was performed, enrolling 17 patients with PSP or CBD, and divided them into four groups to achieve target serum lithium levels of 0.4–0.6, 0.6–0.8, 0.8–1.0, and 1.0–1.2 mmol/L, respectively.[161] Three of the 17 patients were lost to follow-up and were not available to monitor. Out of the remaining 14 patients, 13 withdrew from the study due to lithium side effects. The authors did not report patient side effects as related to the assigned lithium dosage. Thus, this was a failed trial due to the chosen lithium dose being too high for patients to tolerate. These researchers made the same mistake as those who conducted the first lithium AD trial when too high of a lithium dose was chosen, resulting in 14 of the 22 patients withdrawing from the study mostly due to side effects.[162] All that can be gleaned from these studies is that target serum lithium levels greater than 0.6 mmol/L are poorly tolerated in these neurodegenerative diseases. Unfortunately, these studies provide no insight into the tolerability or potential benefits of lower dosages of lithium. As Forlenza et al. and Nunes et al. showed in AD, choosing the correct lithium dosage is critical to the success of a study in neurodegenerative disease.[163]

Multiple system Atrophy (MSA) is another neurodegenerative disease with symptoms similar to PD but with additional symptoms including incoordination and blood pressure fluctuations. The single trial examining the effects of lithium in MSA enrolled nine patients and randomly assigned them to lithium or placebo.[164] Unfortunately, these researchers also made the mistake of setting a very high target serum lithium level of 0.9–1.2 mmol/L, which led to 75% of the lithium-treated patients withdrawing from the study due to side effects. Thus, this was yet another failed trial that provided no useful information on the potential benefits of lower dose lithium therapy.

It should be clear by now that if too high of a lithium dose is used in a neurodegenerative disease clinical trial, it will likely be a failed trial due to unacceptably high patient dropouts. Based on the clinical trials in neurodegenerative diseases reviewed above, a target serum lithium level less than or equal to 0.05 mmol/L provides very good tolerability, may offer benefits to patients' symptoms, and may slow the progression of AD.[165]

Fortunately, the National Institutes of Health have funded a larger randomized controlled trial being conducted at the University of Pittsburgh (the LATTICE study) examining the effects of lithium therapy on both cognition and biomarkers among 80 patients with the pre-AD condition, mild cognitive impairment (MCI).[166] Unfortunately, the lithium dose the researchers chose to study is on the high side (0.6–0.8 mmol/L) and, thus, may be poorly tolerated by the patients. Because MCI patients are less cognitively impaired and younger than AD patients, hopefully the patients will tolerate these higher lithium doses better than AD patients do. This study is currently in progress, and results won't be available until 2024. If there is an unacceptably large number of dropouts in the lithium group due to too high of a dosage being used, this will be yet another missed opportunity to assess lithium's ability to offer hope to AD patients. We will need to wait and see what the LATTICE study shows.

Besides the obstacles that lithium treatment is "too good to be true" and doomed to continue to fail, is there anything else creating headwinds preventing further clinical trial research on lithium? Very likely, it's lithium's stigma.

Lithium's Stigma

As mentioned in Chapter 2, lithium began being used as a medicine in the mid-1800s for treating gout, kidney stones, depression, and general nervousness.[167] In the late 1800s and early 1900s, sodium intake was recognized as a contributor to high blood pressure and heart disease, which gave rise to the use of lithium chloride as a common table salt substitute. Even the popular beverage 7 Up contained lithium in the early 1900s. However, the use of these lithium products was banned in 1949 after the FDA became aware of many cases of lithium toxicity leading to several deaths. Instantly, an element that was believed to be safe enough to use as table salt became known as a poison. It's been an uphill battle for lithium ever since.

Despite ample evidence that lithium was highly effective for treating mania and bipolar disorder, it took until 1970 for the FDA to approve lithium for this indication, making the US the fiftieth country to issue this approval, a delay likely due to lithium's stigma as being a toxic table salt just 20 years earlier. This FDA approval came with the requirement that patients undergo regular serum lithium monitoring because serum lithium levels above the recommended range can cause severe side effects and even death. In addition, about 10% and 32% of patients receiving the proper dosage of lithium for treating bipolar disorder (target serum lithium level 0.6–1.2 mmol/L) can develop low thyroid hormone levels and chronic kidney disease, respectively, necessitating the need for thyroid hormone replacement therapy and/ or lithium therapy discontinuation, respectively.[168] Although use of low-dose lithium therapy (serum lithium level 0.25–0.5 mmol/L) for up to four years in elderly patients was not associated with any change in kidney or thyroid function compared to those receiving placebo, lithium's early history and potential for end-organ toxicities has labeled lithium with the stigma of being a potentially "dangerous drug."[169]

In addition to this stigma, lithium has yet another stigma impeding its repurposing for AD and PD: that lithium is a drug for "crazy people." I hesitate to use the word "crazy" as it has no place in medicine or psychiatry but, truth be told, this is many people's initial thought when hearing about lithium therapy. It's not clear why lithium has this stigma while other drugs FDA-approved for bipolar disorder or depression do not. Even more unfounded, I have heard some people express the concern that taking lithium might *make* them crazy. I believe this knee-jerk misimpression is simply a matter of guilt by association. Because people understand that lithium is a psychiatric medication, this understanding somehow gets mutated into a misunderstanding. I have heard similar concerns from postmenopausal women that I have enrolled into research studies studying the effects of a seizure medication called gabapentin for their hot flashes.[170] Some of these patients asked me if there was a chance that gabapentin might cause them to have seizures. Recurrent seizures, which is called epilepsy, is another condition with unfounded stigmas attached to it, which likely transfer onto the drugs used to treat epilepsy, such as gabapentin. This same unfortunate misunderstanding about lithium likely creates somewhat of a barrier both to patient use of lithium and obtaining funding to research lithium for AD and PD.

It will take some time and much work to chip away at lithium's many stigmas dating back to 1949, but it can be done. How can it be done? It is done with evidence. And how do we gather this evidence? We gather it with clinical trial research like that already performed by Forlenza et al. and Nunes et al.[171]

The Patent Paradox

Another big obstacle to performing clinical trial research is that it is extremely expensive. An estimated cost to enroll 80 patients into a study with MRI scans and biomarker blood tests would be about $3 million. Although government agencies like the National Institutes of Health and private foundations have funded many clinical trials, they have limited funds and resources to distribute. These funding agencies often prefer to fund 10 laboratory studies that may provide new insights into disease mechanisms and therapeutic targets than put all their eggs in one basket and take a risk on a single, very expensive clinical trial that simply gives one of two results: the drug is effective, or it's ineffective. Due to the limited resources available from the government and private foundations, the lion's share of funding for clinical research comes from pharmaceutical companies. But there's a big catch. For a pharmaceutical company to fund clinical research, the drug candidate needs to be under patent protection.

Without a patent, there is virtually no way that a company could make a profit should the drug become FDA approved. This is because after the tens or hundreds of millions of dollars of investments into performing the clinical trials to obtain FDA approval, other companies that make chemically identical generic drugs can almost immediately introduce cheap generics that will prevent insurance companies from paying for the original company's much more expensive drug. Regardless of how promising a drug may be in early testing, like lithium is for AD, pharmaceutical companies will not invest in its development without the prospect of patent protection. Most drugs under patent are completely new molecules synthesized in a laboratory. This clearly is not lithium. Another way for an old drug, like lithium, to obtain patent protection is if a new clinical use is discovered that has never been reported anywhere in the literature or on the internet (i.e., a "new-use patent"). This also is not lithium. One company named Alzamend Neuro has navigated this terrain and obtained a patent for a combination of lithium, proline, and salicylate, which is the active ingredient in aspirin, and is currently investigating this drug combination for treating AD with the hope of gaining FDA approval in the future. It remains to be determined if this company will be successful and if they will be able to defend their patent and effectively ward off generic competition.

As I'm sure you have surmised by this point, I am writing this book because I believe that lithium has great promise for preventing and slowing AD and PD, and I want the world to know about this. And I'm far from the only one with this opinion. Most of the 200-plus articles on lithium referenced in this book conclude with a plea for more research to be performed on these promising applications of lithium. In fact, there have already been two other books written on this topic.[172] But without supporting evidence from clinical trials, the barriers reviewed in this chapter will continue to impede lithium's further development. With the world's largest funders of clinical research (i.e., pharmaceutical companies) largely on the sideline, these barriers are formidable but not insurmountable.

I have personally taken up this effort as a physician-scientist. Over a five-year period, I have prepared and submitted 17 grant applications to major funding agencies in search of support to perform clinical trial research on lithium. Prior to submitting my first lithium grant application, I had much success securing funding from the National Institutes of Health, the most prestigious and discerning funding agency, to support clinical trials in the field of women's health. I mention this to illustrate the strong reluctance funding agencies currently have toward supporting clinical research on lithium that is likely distinct from the quality of the grant applications. I'm glad I have some thick skin and persevered as the fifteenth attempt was finally successful. This small grant was able to support the first clinical trial in PD examining the effects of three different low dosages of lithium on blood-based biomarkers. We will review these results in the next chapter and discuss why positive biomarker study results will be critical to chip away at and ultimately break down the barriers holding up lithium's development.

CHAPTER 5

BIOMARKERS ARE THE KEY

IF YOU HAVE AD OR PD and have Googled research on these diseases, you likely have come across the term "biomarker" several times, which begs the question: what are biomarkers, and why are they so important in our quest to slow AD and PD?

A biomarker is an objective test that reflects a biological process. A good example of a biomarker would be blood glucose (sugar) levels in a patient with diabetes. In this example, blood glucose is both a diagnostic biomarker (meaning that elevated blood glucose is how diabetes is diagnosed) and a therapeutic biomarker (meaning that reducing blood glucose levels with oral medications or insulin reflects the benefits of treatment). With diabetes, use of the blood glucose biomarker is well established and validated to reflect the severity of the disease and the effectiveness of treatments. If patients with diabetes are able to keep their blood glucose levels under good control with daily medication use and exercise, they greatly reduce the long-term medical consequences of having diabetes such as blindness, kidney failure, numbness and pain from nerve damage, blood clots, heart attacks, and strokes. With AD and PD, it's not so straightforward.

Both AD and PD are currently diagnosed based on a patient's symptoms, not based on biomarkers. AD is diagnosed based on a progressive decline in cognitive abilities affecting a person's daily activities, while PD is diagnosed based on the presence of motor symptoms including stiffness, slowness, and tremor. There are several FDA-approved treatments for AD and PD; however, the effectiveness of these treatments is determined by how much the patient's symptoms improve, not by how they affect AD and PD biomarkers. Thus, current AD and PD treatments are called "symptomatic treatments" because they only improve patients' symptoms. It is important to understand that these symptomatic treatments don't do anything to address the underlying disease process that causes these symptoms and causes AD and PD patients to worsen over time. The underlying disease process is the progressive death of brain cells. A treatment that could protect brain cells from dying and slow down the progressive worsening of patients' symptoms would be called a "disease-modifying treatment." This is the huge unmet need in AD and PD. Although a drug called aducanumab was recently FDA-approved as a disease-modifying treatment for AD, the approval was highly controversial, and most experts believe that this drug is ineffective at least based on the currently available data.

In order to confirm that a treatment is "disease-modifying," there would need to be a positive effect on a biomarker that reflects the disease process and not simply a positive effect on patients' symptoms. A good example illustrating this difference would be cancer pain.

Cancerous tumors very often cause pain, which may be a patient's only symptom of the underlying cancer. Improving the patient's pain with morphine will make the patient feel better in the short-term but won't do anything to address what is causing the pain: the underlying growing tumor. On the other hand, administering chemotherapy or radiation treatment may shrink the tumor on an x-ray, which is a biomarker image of the cancer, and objectively confirm that these treatments are addressing the actual cancer itself and not just a symptom of the cancer. Without the x-ray biomarker, it would be very difficult to prove that chemotherapy and radiation are of any benefit to cancer patients simply based on their symptoms. The x-ray biomarker is the key to proving that these treatments are "disease-modifying therapies" for cancer.

Because the fundamental disease process in AD and PD is the progressive death of brain cells, the most logical "disease-progression biomarker" would be a brain imaging technique that reflects the progressive brain damage specific to each disease. Brain atrophy or shrinkage occurs when brain cells die. In AD, brain atrophy in an area called the hippocampus viewed on MRI is a common disease-progression biomarker used in AD clinical trials.[173] In 2019, a different MRI assessment called "free water" that also reflects brain tissue atrophy was shown to better reflect the stages of AD than hippocampal atrophy.[174] When brain cells die or shrink, fluid moves in to occupy the vacancy. This fluid can be measured by MRI and is called free water.[175] As brain cells continue to die, free water levels continue to increase. In PD, increasing levels of free water in brain areas called the substantia nigra (SN) and the thalamus appear to be disease-progression biomarkers similar to how hippocampal free water and atrophy are biomarkers in AD.[176] Thus, if a therapy could be shown to slow hippocampal atrophy and free water accumulation in AD or slow SN and thalamic free water accumulation in PD, such findings would support disease-modifying benefits of the therapy in AD and PD just like chemotherapy and radiation have disease-modifying benefits for cancer by visibly shrinking tumors on x-ray.

Now that you understand the importance of biomarkers for demonstrating a therapy's disease-modifying effects in AD or PD, you will be pleased to learn that there is already such biomarker evidence for lithium therapy in both AD and PD.

Lithium's Effects on AD Biomarkers

Several studies have shown significantly increased hippocampal volume (i.e., reduced hippocampal atrophy) in bipolar disorder patients receiving lithium therapy compared to bipolar patients not receiving lithium and age-matched patients without bipolar disorder.[177] Although these positive neuroimaging biomarker data are from observational studies and not RCTs, they do support possible disease-modifying effects from lithium therapy. These data also support the interpretation that the improved cognition seen in patients with AD and aMCI from lithium therapy in the two Brazilian RCTs reviewed in Chapter 3 was possibly due to a disease-modifying effect and not just a symptomatic effect.[178] If a single RCT could show both improved cognitive symptoms and improved hippocampal volumes and/or free water levels in AD or aMCI, this would be a slam dunk confirming lithium as a disease-modifying therapy. The LATTICE trial that is currently in progress is exactly such an RCT with results expected in 2024.[179] In addition to lithium therapy being associated with reduced hippocampal atrophy,[180] lithium therapy has also been associated with several other favorable neuroimaging outcomes, further supporting its potential disease-modifying effects.[181]

Neuroimaging biomarkers are the most relevant and important type of biomarker for AD and PD; however, they do add complexity and expense to clinical trials. Patients usually need to make additional visits to the study site in order to get the MRI scans, they can become claustrophobic and not be able to tolerate the MRI procedure, and MRI scans are not cheap. Because it has been so challenging for researchers to secure funding to support clinical trials on lithium in AD or PD, several trials have instead focused on assessing blood-based or CSF-based biomarkers, such as the Forlenza et al. trial, to reduce the cost and complexity of biomarker assessment.[182]

How about PD? Are there any clinical trials in PD showing lithium to improve patients' symptoms as well as neuroimaging, CSF, or blood-based biomarkers? The answer is yes, but not in a single trial like that performed by Forlenza et al. in aMCI.

PD Clinical Trial Biomarker Results

The first such report of potential symptomatic benefits from low-dose lithium therapy was a case series that I published based on my own PD patients' experiences, which was reviewed in Chapter 3.[183] Although it is interesting that lithium may be able to improve the symptom of motor fluctuations in PD patients, it doesn't provide any insight into whether lithium can slow down the progressive death of brain cells and the consequent progressive worsening of symptoms in PD. In order to show such "disease-modifying" actions of a drug, as we just reviewed, lithium would need to show positive effects on relevant PD biomarkers. Fortunately, this is exactly what the second study showed.

In this pilot clinical trial (pilot meaning a small exploratory trial) performed at the University at Buffalo, 16 PD patients were randomly assigned to high-, medium-, or low-dose lithium therapy for six months. Three additional PD patients served as controls for comparison purposes and did not receive any lithium therapy for six months. The five patients in the "high-dose" group received lithium carbonate titrated to achieve a serum lithium level of 0.4–0.5 mmol/L. The six patients in the medium-dose group and the five patients in the low-dose group received 45 mg/day and 15 mg/day, respectively, of elemental lithium from OTC lithium aspartate. Blood-based biomarkers were assessed at baseline, three months, and six months.

As reviewed in Chapter 4, it took 15 grant applications over a five-year period to secure a small grant to support this pilot PD clinical trial. In addition, the Department of Neurology at the University at Buffalo received a small donation from a PD patient in the 1990s that was given to support a promising PD research project. Combining these two small funds, we had just enough to cover the costs of assessing the blood-based biomarkers in 19 patients and MRI scans in seven of these 19 patients. It certainly would have been preferable to have enrolled more patients and assessed MRIs on all of them, but the funding constraints limited us to this design.

The two blood-biomarkers of greatest interest were Nurr1 gene expression levels in circulating white blood cells and blood plasma alpha-synuclein levels. In mice, changes in white blood cell gene expression reflect similar changes occurring in the brain.[184] Plasma alpha-synuclein levels are increased in PD likely due to leakage out of the brain and into the bloodstream.[185] As noted in Chapter 3, Nurr1 is a transcription factor that controls the expression of a set of genes that are essential for dopamine brain cell maintenance and survival. Experimental models have shown that when Nurr1 levels are depressed, brain cells become vulnerable to insults and die.[186] Nurr1 levels decrease in the brain by 46% with aging,[187] which is the main risk factor for both AD and PD, and are decreased by about 65% in AD and PD brain and 62% in PD white blood cells compared to people of similar age without AD or PD.[188] One of the genes under the control of Nurr1 is called superoxide dismutase-1 (SOD1). SOD1 is an important enzyme inside brain cells that neutralizes free radicals and, thus, reduces oxidative stress. Nurr1 also decreases the expression of alpha-synuclein and reduces inflammation from microglia.[189] Thus, increasing Nurr1 expression alone can reduce all three points of the Brain's Bermuda Triangle in AD and PD (Figure 1, Chapter 1). In experiments on brain-like cells called PC12 cells, lithium increased Nurr1 by about 180% and protected the cells from pesticide-induced death.[190] Due to all of these findings, Nurr1 has been a promising AD and PD therapeutic target for over 25 years.[191] Any therapy that could increase Nurr1 levels could potentially protect brain cells from dying and slow PD and AD progression.

At the start of this study, I was hoping that lithium therapy would increase white blood cell Nurr1 expression by 200%. Anything above that amount would be a bonus. The results far exceeded my hopes. This pilot study showed that white blood cell Nurr1 levels increased by 420%, 679%, 93%, and 139% in the high-, medium-, and low-dose lithium groups and control group, respectively, after six months of lithium therapy. Because it was previously shown that a 180% increase in Nurr1 protected neuronal cells from toxin-induced death, this pilot clinical trial defined a "Nurr1 responder" as having a six-month Nurr1 increase of more than 200%.[192] With this definition, the Nurr1 responder rates were 20%, 75%, 20%, and 0% for the high-, medium-, and low-dose lithium groups and control group, respectively. Patients' average serum lithium levels at six months were 1,282, 828, 195, and 0.73 micrograms/L, respectively. In addition, white blood cell SOD1 increased by 18%, 127%, -1%, and 8%, respectively, and by 125% and -21% in Nurr1 responders and nonresponders, respectively, after six months. Lithium did not affect plasma alpha-synuclein levels. Thus, the medium-dose lithium group (45 mg/day of lithium aspartate) showed the most robust engagement of the PD therapeutic targets Nurr1 and SOD1 and also had the greatest Nurr1-responder rate.

In addition to the very promising Nurr1 results, the MRI results were even more promising. As reviewed earlier in this chapter, previous studies have shown that "free water" (FW) measured by MRI reflects the site-specific progressive brain cell damage responsible for the progressive worsening of both motor and cognitive symptoms in PD.[193] The site known to be most responsible for the worsening motor symptoms of stiffness, slowness, and tremor in PD is the substantia nigra (SN) where

FW is known to progressively increase over time.[194] The brain sites involved with cognition that show progressive increases in FW over time and best reflect cognitive decline in PD are the dorsomedial nucleus of the thalamus (DMN-T) and the nucleus basalis of Meynert (nbM).[195] Based on these findings, it is likely that a therapy that could slow the progressive increases in FW over time in the SN, DMN-T, and nbM would also slow the progressive worsening of motor and cognitive symptoms in PD. In other words, such a therapy would represent a disease-modifying therapy by slowing down the underlying progressive brain cell damage in PD instead of simply masking the symptoms that result from this brain cell damage.

Out of the seven patients who received MRIs at the start and end of the study, six had reliable MRI data to evaluate at both time points. Two of these patients received high-dose, two received medium-dose, and two received low-dose lithium therapy. When this study began, I was hoping that six months of lithium therapy would be associated with stable or just slight increases in FW in the SN, DMN-T, and nbM over time. What the MRI data showed was much better than what I had hoped. Among the four patients in the high- and medium-dose lithium groups, there were average *decreases* in FW over time in each site, which is the exact opposite of what is known to happen to FW over time in PD.[196] The percent of these four PD patients showing *decreases* in FW in the SN, DMN-T, and nbM were 75%, 50%, and 75%, respectively. For comparison, it is known that in PD patients not receiving lithium, 38%, 13%, and 22% show decreasing FW levels in the SN, DMN-T, and nbM, respectively (unpublished data from our research team at the University at Buffalo). Thus, two to three times as many PD patients receiving high- or medium-dose lithium therapy for six months showed improvements in MRI biomarkers as would be expected based on the natural history of such MRI changes in PD. Decreasing FW implies that the brain cells in these locations are becoming healthier and enlarging and/or sustaining less damage from inflammation over time.[197] The two patients in the low-dose lithium group who received MRIs had increasing FW in the DMN-T and SN but decreasing FW in the nbM. Although it would be unwise to get too excited about promising MRI findings derived from only four patients, they do support a potential disease-modifying effect from high- or medium-dose lithium therapy in concert with the blood-based biomarker results, and the findings clearly justify further clinical trial research on lithium in PD.

In terms of patient side effects, two of the six patients (33%) assigned to medium-dose lithium withdrew from the study, both due to side effects of mental fogginess and sedation. No other side effects were reported by the other 14 patients receiving lithium. One of the two patients who withdrew from the medium-dose group subsequently resumed lithium aspartate but at a reduced dose of 30 mg/day instead of 45 mg/day and reported no associated side effects. After increasing the dose to 45 mg/day, this patient again experienced side effects of mental fogginess and sedation, which resolved when reducing the dose back to 30 mg/day. This patient's serum lithium level at 30 mg/day was less than 0.1 mmol/L.

In summary, this pilot study showed medium-dose OTC lithium aspartate therapy (i.e., 45 mg/day) to most strongly engage the PD blood-based therapeutic targets of Nurr1 and

SOD1 but to be poorly tolerated in one-third of patients despite having serum lithium levels 35% lower than the high-dose lithium carbonate group. Assuming that these findings are reliable and understanding that lithium's side effects are dose-dependent, these findings suggest that lithium aspartate may have greater biological activity at a lower serum lithium level than lithium carbonate; however, it is not clear why this would be. In addition, both high-dose and medium-dose lithium therapy were also associated with decreasing FW levels in the SN, DMN-T, and nbM brain sites, supporting its potential disease-modifying effects in PD. The results of this pilot lithium PD clinical trial will be presented as a poster at the International Congress of Parkinson's Disease and Movement Disorders in Madrid, Spain in September 2022 and submitted for publication in a peer-reviewed medical journal.

Considering the evidence supporting Nurr1 as a promising PD therapeutic target and FW as a valid disease-progression biomarker in PD, the results of this pilot study are highly encouraging and merit further clinical research to identify the lithium dosage and formulation that is well tolerated, that maximally engages PD therapeutic targets, and that significantly reduces brain FW progression over time. If these results can be confirmed in a future randomized controlled trial of much larger size, such data would strongly support lithium as a disease-modifying treatment for PD that would slow PD progression and improve PD prognosis.

The decades of barriers to repurposing lithium for slowing the progression of AD and PD may be close to being toppled. The LATTICE trial results will reportedly be available in 2024, which may provide strong evidence supporting the use of lithium in aMCI patients who are at high risk for AD.[198] I hope that a PD clinical trial with a design very similar to LATTICE, but using a lower lithium dosage, will soon be funded and also show positive results. Recurring waves of positive data from well-designed clinical trials that include neuroimaging data will surely erode the barriers that have impeded further lithium research and move the needle on lithium's acceptance as a repurposed treatment for AD and PD.

Follow Your Nose, It Always Knows

Assuming the day finally arrives when lithium is shown to be a disease-modifying therapy for AD and/or PD, who would stand to benefit the most from it? The answer exists in the meanings of the aphorisms cited in the Introduction and in Chapter 3: TIME IS BRAIN, and "an ounce of prevention is worth a pound of cure." If lithium was proven to be a disease-modifying therapy in AD and PD, starting lithium therapy as soon as possible in those found to be at high risk for developing these conditions would be the most effective strategy to prevent or greatly delay the future onset of AD or PD and would provide the greatest improvements for these patients' futures.

Most everyone is familiar with the standard practice of screening people for high blood pressure or high cholesterol in order to identify those who can benefit from lifestyle modifications and medications in order to prevent them from having a heart attack or stroke in the future. With cardiovascular disease, it is fairly straightforward to screen the population for these cardiovascular risk factors/biomarkers using a blood pressure cuff and a simple blood test. It is also important from a health care cost perspective that these screening tests are easy to administer and are inexpensive.

Wouldn't it be nice if there was a simple and cheap test that could identify patients at risk for future AD or PD? Guess what? There is.

It's a simple and cheap scratch-and-sniff smell test to detect if a person has odor identification deficits. In Chapter 1, we reviewed how in both AD and PD, the disease processes of accumulating sticky proteins, inflammation, and oxidative stress start very early in the part of the brain called the olfactory bulb, which leads to patients slowly developing a decreased sense of smell years before they qualify for a diagnosis of AD or PD. In other words, a decreased sense of smell represents a clinical biomarker that the disease process of AD or PD may have already commenced. Often, this decline in smell is so subtle and slow over many years that patients don't even notice it. But these smell deficits are very apparent if a person takes a validated scratch-and-sniff test such as the Brief Smell Identification Test.[199] If a person sees that their sense of smell is below where it should be or is progressively worsening year after year, this person is likely at significantly higher risk of developing AD or PD in the future. Such a person would then qualify for further testing in order to better stratify their level of risk. If this person was determined to be at "significant risk," however that becomes defined, they would stand to benefit the greatest from daily lithium supplementation (again, assuming that the results from LATTICE and similar PD trials are positive). Anyone concerned about AD or

PD can perform this scratch-and-sniff test at home as it can be purchased online with instant results available.[200]

It will take many more years, perhaps decades, before the field of neurodegenerative disease screening is developed to the point where cardiovascular disease is today. The wonderful thing about low-dose lithium therapy is that people with AD or PD or people at risk for AD or PD don't need to wait decades for all of this development to occur. Low-dose lithium is currently available as an over-the-counter (OTC) dietary supplement in two forms: lithium aspartate and lithium orotate.

This book has introduced you to a wealth of knowledge and has hopefully helped you see the pieces of the puzzle come together not only for what causes AD and PD but also why lithium is a highly promising therapy to prevent and slow these conditions. Now that this story is over and the puzzle is as complete as it can be, for the time being, you probably are asking yourself one final question: should I take OTC lithium supplements?

CHAPTER 6

SHOULD I TAKE OVER-THE-COUNTER LITHIUM SUPPLEMENTS?

LET'S START WITH a simple answer to this question: it's up to you.

This may not be the answer you're looking for, but it's the truth. The information in this book has now empowered you to be able to make your own informed decision. Perhaps you wish to wait for more clinical research to be completed on lithium's use in AD or PD before deciding. This is a completely logical decision. On the other hand, perhaps you have been diagnosed with AD or PD, and the information in this book has convinced you to try over-the-counter (OTC) lithium supplements with the hope that it will slow down your disease and preserve your future while awaiting results from future lithium research studies. If you fall into the latter category, there are some additional things you should know before purchasing OTC lithium.

Lithium is Not FDA-Approved for Treating AD or PD

First of all, don't expect to find a brand of OTC lithium at a vitamin store or on the internet with a label stating that it will prevent or treat AD or PD. You won't. Only the FDA can make "disease claims" regarding a treatment's influence on any disease including AD and PD. The FDA does not review or regulate OTC vitamins, minerals, or dietary supplements. When the FDA approves a prescription medication to treat a disease, the public can have a high degree of confidence that the medication is safe and effective for that indication based on a multitude of both animal and human clinical trial data submitted to the FDA by the sponsoring pharmaceutical company. Because of the enormous expense and complexity of obtaining FDA approval for indications like AD or PD and the inability of lithium to be patented (see Chapter 4), it's doubtful that lithium will ever be FDA approved for treating or preventing AD or PD regardless of the strength of the evidence. Nevertheless, vitamins and dietary supplements available OTC may be effective for preventing or treating diseases; however, their labels cannot state such claims. Such products can only make "structure and function" health claims such as "supports brain health" or "maintains immune cell function."

Lithium's Safety Depends on the Dose

Second of all, as discussed in Chapter 4, long-term use of high-dose lithium can cause kidney damage and thyroid gland suppression. The higher the lithium dose and the longer the duration of use, the greater the chance for organ toxicities. For example, high-dose lithium therapy (an elemental lithium dose of about 160–400 mg/day) for more than 10 years is associated with an increased risk for chronic kidney disease; however, lower-dose lithium therapy (an elemental lithium dose of about 80–200 mg/day) for up to four years is not (Table 4).[201] In addition, lithium therapy can suppress thyroid gland function, sometimes necessitating the need for daily thyroid hormone replacement therapy with a medication like levothyroxine. Fortunately, if lithium-induced thyroid or kidney dysfunction occur, they usually fully resolve after stopping lithium, especially when detected early. In the pilot lithium PD clinical trial reviewed in Chapter 5, there were no meaningful changes in thyroid or kidney function tests after six months of therapy with any of the three low-dosages of lithium therapy tested (Table 4).

Table 4: Lithium Dosage, Serum Level, and Possible Organ Toxicities

Lithium Formulation	Elemental Lithium Dosage	Serum Lithium Range	Known Potential Organ Toxicities
Lithium Carbonate (prescription)	About 160–400 mg/day	0.6–1.2 mmol/L	Possible kidney damage, thyroid gland suppression[202]
Lithium Carbonate (prescription)	About 80–200 mg/day for 4 years	0.25–0.5 mmol/L	None[203]
Lithium Aspartate OTC	45 mg/day for 6 months	0.05–0.16 mmol/L*	None*
Lithium Aspartate OTC	15 mg/day for 6 months	0.01–0.05 mmol/L*	None*

OTC: over-the-counter. *Assessed from the pilot lithium/PD clinical trial.

Remember that you should let your doctor know about any OTC vitamins or supplements you are taking including OTC lithium. When you mention to your doctor that you read this book stating that OTC lithium supplementation may prevent and slow AD and PD, expect a look on your doctor's face that will be some combination of shock, disbelief, and amusement. If you read about all of the barriers holding up lithium's clinical development for AD and PD in Chapter 4, in particular the stigma that is attached to lithium therapy, your doctor's facial expression should come as no surprise. That knee-jerk reaction is common and understandable when people hear about lithium for these nonpsychiatric uses. Also, I can almost guarantee that your doctor will never have heard about lithium's potential to prevent and slow AD and PD and will not be familiar with any of the data detailed in Chapters 2 and 3. In fact, I didn't know any of this valuable information eight years ago before my PD patient Ted told me about the unexpected improvements he experienced after starting lithium and I began reading about lithium. And I'm a movement disorder neurologist who specializes in the treatment of PD!

It will take time to educate the medical community and the population in general as to the potential for low-dose lithium therapy to prevent and slow AD and PD. In the meantime, if your doctor voices concern about your taking OTC lithium, the most important piece of information for you to provide is that OTC lithium is supplied in a much lower dose (5 mg capsules) than what is prescribed to bipolar disease patients (about 300 mg/day of elemental lithium). As a result, the studies performed to date and summarized in Table 4 have shown chronic low-dose lithium therapy to be safe. In addition, you can always bring in your book to show to your doctor, specifically Tables 4 and 5. You very well may find your doctor's facial expression to then change to a look of intrigue and curiosity. The information in this book will be your best advocate in obtaining your doctor's approval to take OTC lithium.

Lithium Orotate or Lithium Aspartate?

If you do decide to take OTC lithium and search for it in vitamin stores or on the internet, you will see there are two OTC lithium products currently available: lithium orotate and lithium aspartate. Does one lithium formulation have any advantages over the other?

I asked myself this same question when designing the pilot lithium PD clinical trial discussed in Chapter 5. Two questions came to mind when considering this decision: 1) does one formulation get absorbed better across the gut in humans and is it, thus, more "bioavailable" for entry into the brain? And 2) are there any safety concerns with either orotate or aspartate as a salt carrier of lithium?

In order to answer the first question, I performed a bit of an experiment on myself. At 6:00 a.m. on three consecutive Monday mornings, I took an equivalent amount of lithium in the forms of lithium carbonate (which is prescription lithium), OTC lithium aspartate, or OTC lithium orotate on an empty stomach. Exactly 1.5 hours after taking the lithium, I had my blood serum lithium level checked. I picked 1.5 hours as that is usually how long it takes for lithium to peak in the bloodstream after taking an oral dose. Both lithium orotate and lithium aspartate list their lithium content in terms of elemental lithium with each capsule containing 5 mg of elemental lithium. Lithium carbonate is labeled according to the full weight of both the lithium and the carbonate components in each pill. For every molecule of lithium carbonate, only 18.8% of the weight is from the elemental lithium with the other 81.2% being from the carbonate component. Thus, 300 mg of lithium carbonate contains 56.4 mg of elemental lithium.

For this experiment, I took 300 mg of lithium carbonate (i.e., 56.4 mg of elemental lithium), 60 mg of elemental lithium from lithium orotate, or 60 mg of elemental lithium from lithium aspartate (i.e., twelve 5 mg capsules). My lithium serum levels 1.5 hours after taking each formulation were 0.3, 0.3, and 0.4 mmol/L, respectively. Therefore, each formulation had about the same absorption across the gut into the bloodstream with perhaps a slight edge in favor of lithium aspartate. Of course, I can't be certain that the results from my experiment generalize to most other adults, but that wasn't the purpose of this experiment. I wanted to make sure that there were not any large differences in absorption among the different formulations of lithium and confirm that OTC lithium actually contained roughly the amount of lithium that was stated on the label.

Now that I was confident that OTC lithium orotate and aspartate actually contained absorbable lithium in the correct doses listed on the labels, I also wondered if one lithium formulation may have a better ability to cross the blood-brain barrier (BBB) and have greater access into brain cells. As reviewed in Chapter 2, the BBB is a formidable barrier that is highly effective for keeping most drugs out of the brain. Once lithium dissociates from its carrier salt (i.e., carbonate, orotate, or aspartate) in the bloodstream, it easily crosses the BBB and brain cells' plasma membranes by hitching a ride with sodium through sodium channels.[204] However, it is not clear how much lithium remains attached to its salt carrier in the bloodstream, which would influence the amount of free lithium available to cross the BBB. Two studies conducted in rats have addressed this very question.

The first study examined blood and brain lithium levels after administering the same dose of either lithium orotate, lithium carbonate, or lithium chloride orally or by injection.[205] This study showed blood and brain lithium levels to be almost identical regardless of the lithium formulation administered or whether it was administered orally or by injection. The results were unchanged whether lithium was administered as a single dose or daily in the rat feed for 20 days. On the other hand, a subsequent similar study showed higher blood and brain lithium levels from a single injection of high dose lithium orotate versus lithium carbonate.[206] Because OTC lithium supplementation is administered orally and not by injection, the current evidence indicates that different oral lithium formulations likely have equivalent abilities to cross the BBB and enter brain cells. These studies did not assess lithium aspartate.

The final question I had was regarding the safety of orotate versus aspartate. The answer to this question turned out to be more revealing than the previous bioavailability questions and ultimately led to the choice of lithium aspartate over lithium orotate for use in our pilot PD clinical trial.

Orotate is a natural compound found in many dairy products and is also synthesized in the body. Because orotate is a natural compound, I was surprised by what I found upon searching on the safety of orotate use. Several studies in rat cancer models have shown short-term daily oral orotate supplementation to increase liver, breast, kidney, small intestine, and lung cancer occurrences.[207] The human orotate dosage equivalent to what dosage increased cancer occurrence in these rat studies was about 9,072 mg/day. The amount of orotate in 45 mg of lithium orotate is 1,130mg (lithium orotate contains about 3.83% elemental lithium). I wondered if a daily orotate dose that is only 12% the dose shown to increase cancer in rats could increase cancer in humans? This is a difficult question to answer with any degree of certainty. However, with cancer, sometimes long-term exposure to very low doses of carcinogens can increase cancer occurrence. For example, it is well known that there is an increased risk of lung cancer in those exposed to secondhand smoke, despite the fact that the daily exposure dose is far less than what smokers inhale.[208] People taking OTC lithium to hopefully prevent or slow down AD or PD would likely take it for many years, perhaps even decades. The rat cancer studies showing tumor-promoting effects from high daily doses of orotate were of short duration. Because of the remote possibility that long-term daily orotate intake could increase cancer in humans, even at 12% the dose shown to increase cancer in rats, I decided that lithium aspartate would likely be a safer choice for our studies as long as there were no safety concerns with daily aspartate intake.

Aspartate, like orotate, is also a natural compound. Aspartate is a nonessential amino acid, meaning that our bodies can produce aspartate from other amino acids, and we are not dependent on a daily supply from our diet. Amino acids are the building blocks of protein and are in most of the foods that we ingest every day. In addition to being an amino acid found in protein, aspartate also functions as an excitatory neurotransmitter in the brain. Neurotransmitter activity enables brain cells to communicate with each other. Some neurotransmitters excite while others inhibit other brain cells. It is known that excessive excitatory neurotransmitter activity in the brain can lead to brain cell damage and death. This has led some to postulate that lithium aspartate should be avoided due to the aspartate component potentially causing excitotoxic brain cell death.[209] While it is true that too much aspartate in the brain can cause excitotoxic brain cell death, I wondered if there was any evidence that administering large aspartate doses to adult rodents could lead to brain damage similar to how large orotate doses led to increased cancer occurrences.

A single study was performed in adult mice to examine for brain toxicity from a systemic injection of high dose aspartate.[210] This study showed that an injection of a human dose equivalent of 35,000 mg of aspartate led to memory impairment and brain cell damage in one part of the brain called the hypothalamus but no other brain sites examined. However, this same study showed that an injection of a human dose equivalent of 28,000 mg of aspartate led to no memory impairment and no brain cell damage to any brain site including the hypothalamus in the adult mice. Lithium aspartate OTC usually contains 4.8% elemental lithium, meaning that a 45 mg dose of elemental lithium from lithium aspartate contains 893mg of aspartate. Thus, the maximum dose of lithium aspartate that was studied in the pilot lithium/PD clinical trial (45 mg/day) contained only 3% of the highest aspartate dose (i.e., 893/28,000) shown *not* to cause any memory impairment or brain cell damage in adult mice. Based on the principles of toxicology, it is highly unlikely that 3% of a nontoxic, one-time dose could cause toxicity when administered daily. For these reasons, lithium aspartate was felt to be a potentially safer OTC lithium formulation to study in our pilot PD clinical trial compared to lithium orotate.

What Dosage Should I Take?

If after taking into consideration all of the potential benefits and risks, you have decided to take OTC lithium supplementation, the final question is what the best dose is to take every day. Unfortunately, there still is no definitive answer to this question, but there is much information to be aware of when making your decision. First of all, there is evidence that a dose as low as 0.06 mg/day or as high as 160–400 mg/day of elemental lithium may be effective for preventing and slowing AD and PD (see Table 5). There is also recent anecdotal evidence suggesting that just 5 mg/day may provide benefits to memory, cognition, and energy levels that are noticeable to patients, which will be reviewed in a few pages.

Table 5: Reported Benefits for AD or PD Associated with Different Lithium Dosages

Elemental Lithium Dosage	Serum Lithium Range	Type of Research Study	Reported Benefits and Side Effects
0.06 mg/day	?	Observational study showing lower rates of AD in municipalities with high drinking water lithium content	22% reduced rate of AD[211]
0.3 mg/day	?	Randomized controlled clinical trial (*n*=110)	Significantly slowed rate of cognitive decline in AD[212]
0.3 mg/day inhaled in a pack-per-day smoker	?	Observational studies	77% reduced rate of PD[213]
Lithium aspartate 45 mg/day	0.05–0.16 mmol/L*	Randomized unblinded clinical trial (*n*=16)	Increased Nurr1 and SOD1 PD therapeutic targets. Reduced PD brain MRI changes (*n*=4). Side effects in 33% of patients.
Lithium carbonate 80–200 mg/day	0.25–0.5 mmol/L	Randomized controlled clinical trial (*n*=45)	Significantly less cognitive decline and improved CSF biomarker in aMCI[214]
Lithium carbonate 160–400 mg/day	0.6–1.2 mmol/L	Observational study	70% reduced rate of AD[215]

*Assessed from the pilot lithium/PD clinical trial.

AD: Alzheimer's disease; PD: Parkinson's disease; aMCI: amnestic Mild Cognitive Impairment (a frequent precursor to AD); CSF: cerebrospinal fluid; Nurr1: nuclear receptor-related 1 protein; SOD1: superoxide dismutase type-1.

The uncertainty about the best lithium dosage is one of the questions we sought to address in our pilot lithium PD clinical trial, which was reviewed in Chapter 5. That study showed 45 mg/day of lithium aspartate to maximally engage the PD therapeutic targets Nurr1 and SOD1, but also caused mental fogginess and sedation side effects in two of the six patients taking this dose. One of these patients later experienced no side effects at 30 mg/day. Perhaps 30 mg/day would have engaged the Nurr1 and SOD1 therapeutic targets as well as 45 mg/day; however, 30 mg/day was not a dosage that was tested in the pilot lithium PD clinical trial.

Thus, until further clinical research is performed, 30 mg/day is likely the highest OTC lithium dose that should be considered by PD or AD patients as well as the general population in order to minimize the chance for any side effects. In addition, although Nurr1 and SOD1 are important PD therapeutic targets, perhaps there are other targets that were not assessed in this clinical trial that lower dosages of lithium aspartate would have engaged.

Perhaps most importantly, our pilot lithium PD trial showed 45 mg/day of lithium aspartate to be the dosage that maximally reduced brain MRI free water over time, *which is the opposite* of what is known to naturally occur over time in PD. Although the implication of these findings is that lithium aspartate at 45 mg/day may be slowing the progressive damage of brain cells in PD, these data stem from only two PD patients. As stated in Chapter 5, a larger study will need to be performed to determine if these findings are reliable and to determine the optimal lithium aspartate dosage to maximally engage both MRI and blood-based biomarkers. These are all questions that remain to be answered in future PD and AD clinical trials. It also remains to be determined if positive changes in these blood-based and MRI biomarkers associated with lithium therapy are also associated with improvements in symptoms in patients with PD or AD. After all, AD and PD patients want to experience improvements in their symptoms in the short-term and/or know that their symptoms are progressing more slowly over the long-term from taking a therapy. Biomarkers are important, but symptoms are more important to patients. It is very satisfying to actually "feel better" after starting a new treatment.

Speaking about feeling better, you deserve to hear about several patients that have reported noticeable and satisfying improvements in their symptoms after starting OTC lithium therapy at only 5 mg/day. However, before I elaborate on these patients' experiences, understand that such anecdotal cases do not prove anything and should be considered nothing more than interesting observations at this time. Nevertheless, because they have grabbed my attention and suggest that lithium aspartate dosages as low as 5 mg/day may provide noticeable symptomatic benefits, I will share them with you with the understanding that much more research needs to be performed, especially randomized controlled trials (RCTs), to determine if these observations translate into an effective treatment.

The first patient is a 68-year-old man diagnosed with Lewy body dementia two years prior to his starting lithium aspartate at 5 mg/day. Lewy body dementia has some symptoms similar to PD and also progressively worsens over time due to the Brain's Bermuda Triangle (Figure 1, Chapter 1) just like AD and PD; however, these patients also experience problematic cognitive deficits very early in the disease, which was the case with this patient. His wife felt that he had become forgetful, withdrawn, and quieter and had lost his typical sharp wit and sense of humor. He also noticed that his physical performance when playing pickleball had declined substantially. This patient started OTC lithium 5 mg a day with the hope that it may slow the progression of his disease and help to keep him from getting worse than he already was. Surprisingly, within a few weeks of starting OTC lithium 5 mg a day, he said he felt "remarkably better." He reported improved memory, mood, energy, talkativeness, and athleticism while playing pickleball. He also felt like his wit and personality had returned to his "normal self." He said that he used to have mostly bad days and rarely had a good day. After starting lithium, he reported having mostly good days and some mediocre days but no longer had any bad days. He has continued at this level of functioning without any change in medications now for three years, which is unusual for a disease like Lewy body dementia.

The next patient is an 80-year-old woman who had PD for seven years and who started lithium aspartate at 5 mg a day with the hope that it may slow down the progression of her disease. Seven months later, she reported that she and her husband noticed her cognition and mental sharpness had improved, which were unanticipated benefits. She reported she was doing better at her daily crossword puzzles and had improved short-term memory and word-finding abilities. One year later, she was still taking lithium aspartate 5 mg a day and reported these same benefits without any noticeable worsening in her cognition.

The next person is an 82-year-old man diagnosed with PD

for two years who was noticing several cognitive problems. He was becoming more forgetful, would often have difficulty following conversations, and had trouble finding the right word when speaking. He was a retired engineer and banker and was now having difficulty with simple calculations he used to be able to do quickly in his head. About a week after starting lithium aspartate at 5 mg a day, this patient reported that his memory, conversation abilities, and ability to perform calculations were noticeably better. This patient's son said that he witnessed these improvements in his father during a finance board meeting they both attended. Before starting lithium, his father would sit quietly during these meetings and had difficulty following the discussions. After starting lithium, he became eager to participate and was able to perform calculations and recall purchases made five years ago with accuracy. This PD patient has now been taking lithium aspartate 5 mg/day for five months and continues to notice these benefits.

Although these anecdotal cases are promising, the benefits experienced by each of these people may simply represent placebo effects. That is, because these patients were hoping for and anticipating benefit, they indeed experienced benefit from taking a capsule a day regardless of what was in the capsule. As stated several times in this book, the gold-standard method for assessing a therapy's effectiveness is the RCT. The possibility that a low dosage of lithium therapy may improve cognition in patients with Lewy body dementia or PD, as has been shown in AD, will need to be assessed in an RCT.[216]

Considering that the smallest dose available for OTC lithium aspartate capsules is 5 mg, any lithium aspartate dosage between 5 and 45 mg/day is supported by the data summarized in Table 5 as having the potential to prevent and slow AD and PD. Until results from future clinical trials are available, it is very reasonable for AD or PD patients interested in taking lithium aspartate to take only 5 mg/day. For those who wish to try higher dosages, increasing the total daily dose by 5 mg every one to two weeks up to a maximum of 30 mg a day will help to minimize the chance for side effects. If side effects of mental fogginess or sedation occur, the daily lithium dosage should be lowered until the side effects fully resolve. Taking the majority or all of the daily lithium dosage at bedtime may also help to prevent these potential side effects from occurring during the day. Also, people with any known kidney disease or taking diuretic medications (aka "water pills") should talk to their doctor before taking OTC lithium and should likely not take more than 10 mg/day. People with kidney disease or taking diuretics will have higher lithium blood levels and, thus, be more likely to experience side effects if they push the dosage too high.

CONCLUSION

I HOPE THAT YOU NOW see how many different pieces of the AD/ PD treatment puzzle have come together to form a picture of hope. Hope that something as simple as daily dietary supplementation with OTC lithium may prevent and slow AD and PD, providing patients with a brighter future.

You saw in Chapter 1 how the Brain's Bermuda Triangle of spreading sticky proteins, inflammation, and oxidative stress is responsible for the progressive death of brain cells and worsening of symptoms in AD and PD and how the world's most dangerous consumer product, cigarettes, may be teaching us about the benefits of low-dose lithium therapy from as far back as 1959. In Chapter 2, you saw that low-dose lithium effectively targets and quells all three points of the Brain's Bermuda triangle and is highly effective in many animal models of AD and PD. In Chapter 3, you learned about the vast amount of *human* evidence that daily lithium intake, whether from the drinking water supply, prescription lithium for bipolar disorder, or use in randomized controlled trials (RCTs), may prevent and slow AD and PD *in humans*. In Chapter 4, you learned about the headwinds facing the development of lithium into a proven therapy for AD and PD. In Chapter 5, you learned what is needed to overcome these headwinds by performing well-designed RCTs using biomarkers and learned about the promising results of the first PD/lithium biomarker clinical trial ever performed. Finally, in Chapter 6 you learned about the practical information needed to make your own informed decision on whether you should take OTC lithium supplementation, which type of lithium to take—and at what dosage—while awaiting the results of future RCTs, like the ongoing LATTICE trial in AD being funded by the National Institutes of Health (NIH).[217]

Although the LATTICE trial is certainly a step in the right direction, much more research needs to be performed on lithium in AD and PD patients, especially if the LATTICE trial shows an unacceptable level of patient dropouts due to side effects from too high of a lithium dosage being used (reviewed in detail in Chapter 4). The only way for future AD and PD studies to be performed, utilizing many different biomarkers and studying several different lithium dosages, is for research funding to be available. To win this fight and get this research performed, there are some things that you can do right now to help.

First of all, you can share this book with your friends, family, AD/PD support group members, doctors, and social media network and let them all know what you think about the book. You can also share this book's website, PromiseofLithium.com, where anyone can register to receive periodic email updates with results from new lithium research studies and clinical trials. (Emails will never be shared or sold to anyone.) In this way, the educational mission of this book can live on. At the time I wrote this book, there was virtually no one in the world besides a few dozen scientists aware of the great potential that low-dose lithium therapy has to prevent and slow AD and PD. You can change that. You can share your excitement with others. That's why I wrote this book, to share my excitement with you. If you are now excited, too, pass your excitement along. Excitement can be contagious and can supercharge progress. We need more research dollars from the NIH and private foundations to be devoted to supporting lithium clinical trials in AD and PD in order for progress to be made. Your excitement, if passed along, will eventually be noticed by funding agencies and, voilà, progress will be made quickly.

Secondly, you can directly email the directors at the NIH who oversee the grants and distribution of funds at the two institutes that support AD and PD research and request that their institutes support clinical trial research on lithium for AD and PD. Feel free to mention the information that you learned in this book as the reason for your request. The National Institute on Aging (NIA) funds research on AD, and the current director is Richard J. Hodes, MD (hodesr@31.nia.nih.gov). The National Institute of Neurological Disorders and Stroke (NINDS) funds research on PD, and the current director is Walter J. Koroshetz, MD (koroshetzw@mail.nih.gov). The vast majority of research funding in the US is derived from the NIH. Therefore, if you and enough people in your social network email the NIH with this request, we may very well see new NIH grant proposals specifically requesting clinical trial applications on lithium for AD and PD.

Third, if you have the means, you can donate directly to private research funding agencies such as the Alzheimer's Association or the Michael J. Fox Foundation. And when you donate, make a notation that you strongly support the funding of clinical trial research on lithium for AD or PD, respectively. If you want to ensure that your donation is devoted toward clinical trial research on lithium for AD or PD, you can donate to the "Pioneering Researcher Fund" in the Department of Neurology at the University at Buffalo (UB) (https://ubfoundation.buffalo.edu/giving/index.php?gift_allocation=01-3-0-09002), which is a fund under my direction. Once adequate funding is raised, we will first conduct an RCT assessing low-dose lithium aspartate's effects on biomarker progression in PD, including MRI and blood-based biomarkers. If we have adequate funding, we will also spearhead an RCT assessing lithium's effects on biomarker progression in AD, very similar to the ongoing LATTICE trial, but using low dosages of OTC lithium aspartate instead of the higher dosages of prescription lithium carbonate being used in LATTICE. Results from these RCTs will greatly inform patients and the overall medical community as to the benefits of lithium therapy for slowing PD and AD.

Finally, if you decide to take OTC lithium supplementation and notice improvements in any of your symptoms, let your doctors know. Doctors do listen. If you share your experiences, your doctors may get intrigued and curious just like I did in 2014 when Ted and his wife told me their surprising news. The more interest there is in the medical community to advance the research the better. Through research and dialogue, we can collectively make a difference.

Progress is being made in our fight to find treatments to prevent and slow AD and PD. With your new knowledge about AD and PD and hope that OTC lithium supplementation may be an important intervention, you are now in the ring with the world's doctors and researchers who are spearheading these efforts. Welcome to the fight.

ACKNOWLEDGMENTS

I would like to thank all of my patients who have placed their trust in me for their care and have privileged me with observations about their diseases that have made this book possible.

REFERENCES

1 James BD, Leurgans SE, Hebert LE, Scherr PA, Yaffe K, Bennett DA. Contribution of Alzheimer disease to mortality in the United States. *Neurology.* 2014;82(12):1045-50.

2 Hurd MD, Martorell P, Delavande A, Mullen KJ, Langa KM. Monetary costs of dementia in the United States. *N Engl J Med.* 2013;368(14):1326-34.

3 Riedel S. Edward Jenner and the history of smallpox and vaccination. *Proc (Bayl Univ Med Cent).* 2005;18(1):21-25;

   Lind J. *A treatise of the scurvy, in three parts. Containing an inquiry into the nature, causes, and cure, of that disease. Together with a critical and chronological view of what has been published on the subject.* Sands, Murray and Cochran; 1753. https://archive. org/details/b30507054/page/190/mode/2up.

4 Guttuso T Jr, Kurlan R, McDermott MP, Kieburtz K. Gabapentin's effects on hot flashes in postmenopausal women: a randomized controlled trial. *Obstet Gynecol.* 2003;101(2):337-45.

5 Guttuso T Jr, Messing S, Tu X, et al. Effect of gabapentin on hyperemesis gravidarum: a double-blind, randomized controlled trial. *Am J Obstet Gynecol MFM.* 2021;3(1):100273.

6 Braak H, Thal DR, Ghebremedhin E, Del Tredici K. Stages of the pathologic process in Alzheimer disease: age categories from 1 to 100 years. *J Neuropathol Exp Neurol.* 2011;70(11):960-69;

   Braak H, Del Tredici K, Rüb U, de Vos RAI, Jansen Steur ENH, Braak E. Staging of brain pathology related to sporadic Parkinson's disease. *Neurobiol Aging.* 2003;24(2):197-211.

7 Braak H, Thal DR, Ghebremedhin E, Del Tredici K. Stages of the pathologic process in Alzheimer disease: age categories from 1 to 100 years. *J Neuropathol Exp Neurol.* 2011;70(11):960-69;

   Braak H, Del Tredici K, Rüb U, de Vos RAI, Jansen Steur ENH, Braak E. Staging of brain pathology related to sporadic Parkinson's disease. *Neurobiol Aging.* 2003;24(2):197-211;

Moscoso A, Grothe MJ, Ashton NJ, et al. Longitudinal associations of blood phosphorylated tau181 and neurofilament light chain with neurodegeneration in Alzheimer disease. *JAMA Neurol.* 2021;78(4):396-406;

Bierer LM, Hof PR, Purohit DP, et al. Neocortical neurofibrillary tangles correlate with dementia severity in Alzheimer's disease. *Arch Neurol.* 1995;52(1):81-8;

La Joie R, Visani AV, Baker SL, et al. Prospective longitudinal atrophy in Alzheimer's disease correlates with the intensity and topography of baseline tau-PET. *Science Transl Med.* 2020;12.

8   Braak H, Thal DR, Ghebremedhin E, Del Tredici K. Stages of the pathologic process in Alzheimer disease: age categories from 1 to 100 years. *J Neuropathol Exp Neurol.* 2011;70(11):960-69.

9   Braak H, Thal DR, Ghebremedhin E, Del Tredici K. Stages of the pathologic process in Alzheimer disease: age categories from 1 to 100 years. *J Neuropathol Exp Neurol.* 2011;70(11):960-69;

Matchett BJ, Grinberg LT, Theofilas P, Murray ME. The mechanistic link between selective vulnerability of the locus coeruleus and neurodegeneration in Alzheimer's disease. *Acta Neuropathol.* 2021;141(5):631-50.

10   Murphy C. Olfactory and other sensory impairments in Alzheimer disease. *Nat Rev Neurol.* 2019;15(1):11-24.

11   Pamphlett R. Uptake of environmental toxicants by the locus ceruleus: a potential trigger for neurodegenerative, demyelinating and psychiatric disorders. *Med Hypotheses.* 2014;82(1):97-104;

Pamphlett R, Kum Jew S. Uptake of inorganic mercury by human locus ceruleus and corticomotor neurons: implications for amyotrophic lateral sclerosis. *Acta Neuropathol Commun.* 2013;1:1-13;

Cohen Z, Molinatti G, Hamel E. Astroglial and vascular interactions of noradrenaline terminals in the rat cerebral cortex. *J Cereb Blood Flow Metab.* 1997;17(8):894-904;

Paspalas CD, Papadopoulos GC. Ultrastructural relationships between noradrenergic nerve fibers and non-neuronal elements in the rat cerebral cortex. *Glia.* 1996;17(2):133-46.

12   Yoshiyama Y, Higuchi M, Zhang B, et al. Synapse loss and microglial activation precede tangles in a P301S tauopathy mouse model. *Neuron.* 2007;53(3):337-51;

Kitazawa M, Cheng D, Tsukamoto MR, et al. Blocking IL-1 signaling rescues cognition, attenuates tau pathology, and restores neuronal beta-catenin pathway function in an Alzheimer's disease model. *J Immunol.* 2011;187(12):6539-49;

Gao HM, Kotzbauer PT, Uryu K, Leight S, Trojanowski JQ, Lee VM. Neuroinflammation and oxidation/nitration of alpha-synuclein linked to dopaminergic neurodegeneration. *J Neurosci.* 2008;28(30):7687-98;

Kim GH, Kim JE, Rhie SJ, Yoon S. The role of oxidative stress in neurodegenerative diseases. *Exp Neurobiol.* 2015;24(4):325-40.

13 Gottesman RF, Albert MS, Alonso A, et al. Associations between midlife
    vascular risk factors and 25-year incident dementia in the Atherosclerosis Risk in
    Communities (ARIC) cohort. *JAMA Neurol.* 2017;74(10):1246-54.

14 Lennon MJ, Makkar SR, Crawford JD, Sachdev PS. Midlife hypertension and
    Alzheimer's disease: a systematic review and meta-analysis. *J Alzheimers Dis.*
    2019;71(1):307-16.

15 Vagelatos NT, Eslick GD. Type 2 diabetes as a risk factor for Alzheimer's disease:
    the confounders, interactions, and neuropathology associated with this relationship.
    Epidemiol Rev. 2013;35:152-60.

16 Iwagami M, Qizilbash N, Gregson J, et al. Blood cholesterol and risk of dementia
    in more than 1.8 million people over two decades: a retrospective cohort study. *The
    Lancet Healthy Longevity.* 2021;2(8):e498-e506.

17 Cataldo JK, Prochaska JJ, Glantz SA. Cigarette smoking is a risk factor for
    Alzheimer's disease: an analysis controlling for tobacco industry affiliation. *J
    Alzheimers Dis.* 2010;19(2):465-80.

18 Mann CJ. Observational research methods. Research design II: cohort, cross
    sectional, and case-control studies. *Emerg Med J.* 2003;20(1):54-60.

19 Wadley AJ, Veldhuijzen van Zanten JJ, Aldred S. The interactions of oxidative stress
    and inflammation with vascular dysfunction in ageing: the vascular health triad. *Age
    (Dordr).* 2013;35(3):705-18;

    Guzik TJ, Touyz RM. Oxidative stress, inflammation, and vascular aging in
    hypertension. *Hypertension.* 2017;70(4):660-67; Steven S, Frenis K, Oelze M, et al.
    Vascular inflammation and oxidative stress: major triggers for cardiovascular disease.
    Oxid Med Cell Longev. 2019;2019:7092151;

    Conklin DJ, Schick S, Blaha MJ, et al. Cardiovascular injury induced by
    tobacco products: assessment of risk factors and biomarkers of harm. A Tobacco
    Centers of Regulatory Science compilation. *Am J Physiol Heart Circ Physiol.*
    2019;316(4):H801-27;

    Yang X, Li Y, Li Y, et al. Oxidative stress-mediated atherosclerosis: mechanisms and
    therapies. *Front Physiol.* 2017;8:600.

20 van Rooden S, Goos JD, van Opstal AM, et al. Increased number of microinfarcts in
    Alzheimer disease at 7-T MR imaging. *Radiology.* 2014;270(1):205-11;

    Kapasi A, Leurgans SE, Arvanitakis Z, Barnes LL, Bennett DA, Schneider JA. Aβ
    (amyloid beta) and tau tangle pathology modifies the association between small
    vessel disease and cortical microinfarcts. *Stroke.* 2021;52(3):1012-21;

    Koton S, Pike JR, Johansen M, et al. Association of ischemic stroke incidence,
    severity, and recurrence with dementia in the Atherosclerosis Risk in Communities
    cohort study. *JAMA Neurol.* 2022;79(3):271-80.

21 Roberts RO, Christianson TJ, Kremers WK, et al. Association between olfactory
    dysfunction and amnestic mild cognitive impairment and Alzheimer disease
    dementia. *JAMA Neurol.* 2016;73(1):93-101;

Dintica CS, Marseglia A, Rizzuto D, et al. Impaired olfaction is associated with cognitive decline and neurodegeneration in the brain. *Neurology.* 2019;92(7):e700-e709.

22 Yoshiyama Y, Higuchi M, Zhang B, et al. Synapse loss and microglial activation precede tangles in a P301S tauopathy mouse model. *Neuron.* 2007;53(3):337-51;

Kitazawa M, Cheng D, Tsukamoto MR, et al. Blocking IL-1 signaling rescues cognition, attenuates tau pathology, and restores neuronal beta-catenin pathway function in an Alzheimer's disease model. *J Immunol.* 2011;187(12):6539-49;

Gao HM, Kotzbauer PT, Uryu K, Leight S, Trojanowski JQ, Lee VM. Neuroinflammation and oxidation/nitration of alpha-synuclein linked to dopaminergic neurodegeneration. *J Neurosci.* 2008;28(30):7687-98;

Kim GH, Kim JE, Rhie SJ, Yoon S. The role of oxidative stress in neurodegenerative diseases. *Exp Neurobiol.* 2015;24(4):325-40.

23 Kang JH, Irwin DJ, Chen-Plotkin AS, et al. Association of cerebrospinal fluid beta-amyloid 1-42, T-tau, P-tau181, and alpha-synuclein levels with clinical features of drug-naive patients with early Parkinson disease. *JAMA Neurol.* 2013;70(10):1277-87;

Wessels AM, Tariot PN, Zimmer JA, et al. Efficacy and safety of lanabecestat for treatment of early and mild Alzheimer disease: the AMARANTH and DAYBREAK-ALZ randomized clinical trials. *JAMA Neurol.* 2020;77(2):199-209.

24 Nixon RA. The role of autophagy in neurodegenerative disease. *Nat Med.* 2013;19(8):983-97.

25 Cuervo AM, Stefanis L, Fredenburg R, Lansbury PT, Sulzer D. Impaired degradation of mutant alpha-synuclein by chaperone-mediated autophagy. *Science.* 2004;305(5688):1292-95.

26 Gao HM, Kotzbauer PT, Uryu K, Leight S, Trojanowski JQ, Lee VM. Neuroinflammation and oxidation/nitration of alpha-synuclein linked to dopaminergic neurodegeneration. *J Neurosci.* 2008;28(30):7687-98.

27 Yan MH, Wang X, Zhu X. Mitochondrial defects and oxidative stress in Alzheimer disease and Parkinson disease. *Free Radic Biol Med,* 2013;62:90-101.

28 Yoshiyama Y, Higuchi M, Zhang B, et al. Synapse loss and microglial activation precede tangles in a P301S tauopathy mouse model. *Neuron.* 2007;53(3):337-51;

Kitazawa M, Cheng D, Tsukamoto MR, et al. Blocking IL-1 signaling rescues cognition, attenuates tau pathology, and restores neuronal beta-catenin pathway function in an Alzheimer's disease model. *J Immunol.* 2011;187(12):6539-49;

Gao HM, Kotzbauer PT, Uryu K, Leight S, Trojanowski JQ, Lee VM. Neuroinflammation and oxidation/nitration of alpha-synuclein linked to dopaminergic neurodegeneration. *J Neurosci.* 2008;28(30):7687-98;

Kim GH, Kim JE, Rhie SJ, Yoon S. The role of oxidative stress in neurodegenerative diseases. *Exp Neurobiol.* 2015;24(4):325-40; Solleiro-Villavicencio H, Rivas-Arancibia S. Effect of chronic oxidative stress on neuroinflammatory response mediated by CD4 + T cells in neurodegenerative diseases. *Front Cell Neurosci.* 2018;12:114.

29 Gold A, Turkalp ZT, Munoz DG. Enteric alpha-synuclein expression is increased in Parkinson's disease but not Alzheimer's disease. *Mov Disord.* 2013;28(2):237-40.

30 Abbott RD, Petrovitch H, White LR, et al. Frequency of bowel movements and the future risk of Parkinson's disease. *Neurology* 2001;57(3):456-62.

31 Braak H, Del Tredici K, Rüb U, de Vos RAI, Jansen Steur ENH, Braak E. Staging of brain pathology related to sporadic Parkinson's disease. *Neurobiol Aging.* 2003;24(2):197-211;

Fullard ME, Morley JF, Duda JE. Olfactory dysfunction as an early biomarker in Parkinson's disease. *Neurosci Bull.* 2017;33(5):515-25.

32 Roberts RO, Christianson TJ, Kremers WK, et al. Association between olfactory dysfunction and amnestic mild cognitive impairment and Alzheimer disease dementia. *JAMA Neurol.* 2016;73(1):93-101.

33 Aguirre-Mardones C, Iranzo A, Vilas D, et al. Prevalence and timeline of nonmotor symptoms in idiopathic rapid eye movement sleep behavior disorder. *J Neurol.* 2015;262(6):1568-78;

Boeve BF, Saper CB. REM sleep behavior disorder: a possible early marker for synucleinopathies. *Neurology.* 2006;66(6):796-97.

34 Sule RO, Condon L, Gomes AV. A common feature of pesticides: oxidative stress—the role of oxidative stress in pesticide-induced toxicity. *Oxid Med Cell Longev.* 2022;2022:5563759;

Mirowsky JE, Dailey LA, Devlin RB. Differential expression of pro-inflammatory and oxidative stress mediators induced by nitrogen dioxide and ozone in primary human bronchial epithelial cells. *Inhal Toxicol.* 2016;28(8):374-82;

Selemidis S, Seow HJ, Broughton BR, et al. Nox1 oxidase suppresses influenza a virus-induced lung inflammation and oxidative stress. *PLoS One.* 2013;8(4):e60792.

35 Ascherio A, Chen H, Weisskopf MG, et al. Pesticide exposure and risk for Parkinson's disease. *Ann Neurol.* 2006;60(2):197-203.

36 Jo S, Kim YJ, Park KW, et al. Association of NO2 and other air pollution exposures with the risk of Parkinson disease. *JAMA Neurol.* 2021;78(7):800-808.

37 Cocoros NM, Svensson E, Szépligeti SK, et al. Long-term risk of Parkinson disease following influenza and other infections. *JAMA Neurol.* 2021;78(12):1461-70.

38 Mann CJ. Observational research methods. Research design II: cohort, cross sectional, and case-control studies. *Emerg Med J.* 2003;20(1):54-60.

39 van Rooden S, Goos JD, van Opstal AM, et al. Increased number of microinfarcts in Alzheimer disease at 7-T MR imaging. *Radiology.* 2014;270(1):205-11;

Kapasi A, Leurgans SE, Arvanitakis Z, Barnes LL, Bennett DA, Schneider JA. Aβ (amyloid beta) and tau tangle pathology modifies the association between small vessel disease and cortical microinfarcts. *Stroke.* 2021;52(3):1012-21;

Ghebremedhin E, Rosenberger A, Rüb U, et al. Inverse relationship between cerebrovascular lesions and severity of lewy body pathology in patients with lewy body diseases. *J Neuropathol Exp Neurol.* 2010;69(5):442-48.

40 Lennon MJ, Makkar SR, Crawford JD, Sachdev PS. Midlife hypertension and Alzheimer's disease: a systematic review and meta-analysis. *J Alzheimers Dis.* 2019;71(1):307-16.

41 Chen J, Zhang C, Wu Y, Zhang D. Association between hypertension and the risk of Parkinson's disease: a meta-analysis of analytical studies. *Neuroepidemiology.* 2019;52(3-4):181-92.

42 Vagelatos NT, Eslick GD. Type 2 diabetes as a risk factor for Alzheimer's disease: the confounders, interactions, and neuropathology associated with this relationship. *Epidemiol Rev.* 2013;35:152-60.

43 Driver JA, Smith A, Buring JE, Gaziano JM, Kurth T, Logroscino G. Prospective cohort study of type 2 diabetes and the risk of Parkinson's disease. *Diabetes Care.* 2008;31(10):2003-5.

44 Iwagami M, Qizilbash N, Gregson J, et al. Blood cholesterol and risk of dementia in more than 1.8 million people over two decades: a retrospective cohort study. *The Lancet Healthy Longevity.* 2021;2(8):e498-e506.

45 Jiang Z, Xu X, Gu X, et al. Effects of higher serum lipid levels on the risk of Parkinson's disease: a systematic review and meta-analysis. *Front Neurol.* 2020;11:597.

46 Cataldo JK, Prochaska JJ, Glantz SA. Cigarette smoking is a risk factor for Alzheimer's disease: an analysis controlling for tobacco industry affiliation. *J Alzheimers Dis.* 2010;19(2):465-80.

47 Ritz B, Ascherio A, Checkoway H, et al. Pooled analysis of tobacco use and risk of Parkinson disease. *Arch Neurol.* 2007;64(7):990-97.

48 Mann CJ. Observational research methods. Research design II: cohort, cross sectional, and case-control studies. *Emerg Med J.* 2003;20(1):54-60.

49 Csiszar A, Podlutsky A, Wolin MS, Losonczy G, Pacher P, Ungvari Z. Oxidative stress and accelerated vascular aging: implications of cigarette smoking. *Front Biosci (Landmark Ed).* 2009;14(8):3128-44.

50 Dorn HF. Tobacco consumption and mortality from cancer and other diseases. *Public Health Rep (1896).* 1959;74(7):581-93.

51 Ritz B, Ascherio A, Checkoway H, et al. Pooled analysis of tobacco use and risk of Parkinson disease. *Arch Neurol.* 2007;64(7):990-97;

Li X, Li W, Liu G, Shen X, Tang Y. Association between cigarette smoking and Parkinson's disease: a meta-analysis. *Arch Gerontol Geriatr.* 2015;61(3):510-16.

52 Gallo V, Vineis P, Cancellieri M, et al. Exploring causality of the association between smoking and Parkinson's disease. *Int J Epidemiol.* 2018;48(3):912-25;

Liu W, Wang B, Xiao Y, Wang D, Chen W. Secondhand smoking and neurological disease: a meta-analysis of cohort studies. *Rev Environ Health.* 2020;36(2):271-77.

53 Morozova N, O'Reilly EJ, Ascherio A. Variations in gender ratios support the connection between smoking and Parkinson's disease. *Mov Disord.* 2008;23(10):1414-19.

54 Dorsey ER, Sherer T, Okun MS, Bloem BR. The emerging evidence of the Parkinson pandemic. *J Parkinsons Dis.* 2018;8(s1):S3-S8.

55 Tanner CM, Goldman SM, Aston DA, et al. Smoking and Parkinson's disease in twins. *Neurology.* 2002;58(4):581-88;

Wirdefeldt K, Gatz M, Pawitan Y, Pedersen NL. Risk and protective factors for Parkinson's disease: a study in Swedish twins. *Ann Neurol.* 2005;57(1):27-33.

56 Tsuang D, Larson EB, Li G, et al. Association between lifetime cigarette smoking and Lewy body accumulation. *Brain Pathol.* 2010;20(2):412-18;

Chang RC, Ho YS, Wong S, Gentleman SM, Ng HK. Neuropathology of cigarette smoking. *Acta Neuropathol.* 2014;127(1):53-69.

57 Talhout R, Schulz T, Florek E, van Benthem J, Wester P, Opperhuizen A. Hazardous compounds in tobacco smoke. *Int J Environ Res Public Health.* 2011;8(2):613-28.

58 Quik M, Perez XA, Bordia T. Nicotine as a potential neuroprotective agent for Parkinson's disease. *Mov Disord.* 2012;27(8):947-57.

59 Oertel W, Müller H, Schade-Brittinger C, et al. The NIC-PD-study—a randomized, placebo-controlled, double-blind, multi-centre trial to assess the disease-modifying potential of transdermal nicotine in early Parkinson's disease in Germany and N. America [abstract]. *Mov Disord.* 2018;33(suppl 2).

60 Oertel W, Müller H, Schade-Brittinger C, et al. The NIC-PD-study—a randomized, placebo-controlled, double-blind, multi-centre trial to assess the disease-modifying potential of transdermal nicotine in early Parkinson's disease in Germany and N. America [abstract]. *Mov Disord.* 2018;33(suppl 2).

61 Athauda D, Foltynie T. The ongoing pursuit of neuroprotective therapies in Parkinson disease. *Nat Rev Neurol.* 2015;11(1):25-40;

Olanow CW, Kieburtz K, Schapira AH. Why have we failed to achieve neuroprotection in Parkinson's disease? *Ann Neurol.* 2008;64(suppl 2):S101-10.

62 Lähteenvuo M, Tanskanen A, Taipale H, et al. Real-world effectiveness of pharmacologic treatments for the prevention of rehospitalization in a Finnish nationwide cohort of patients with bipolar disorder. *JAMA Psychiatry.* 2018;75(4):347-55.

63 Jathar VS, Pendharkar PR, Pandey VK, et al. Manic depressive psychosis in India and the possible role of lithium as a natural prophylactic. II—Lithium content of diet and some biological fluids in Indian subjects. *J Postgrad Med.* 1980;26(1):39-44.

64 Guttuso T Jr, Russak E, De Blanco MT, Ramanathan M. Could high lithium levels in tobacco contribute to reduced risk of Parkinson's disease in smokers? *J Neurol Sci.* 2019;397:179-80.

65 Coffey CE, Ross DR, Ferren EL, Sullivan JL, Olanow CW. Treatment of the "on-off" phenomenon in Parkinsonism with lithium carbonate. *Ann Neurol.* 1982;12:375-79.

66 Coffey CE, Ross DR, Massey EW, Olanow CW. Dyskinesias associated with lithium therapy in parkinsonism. *Clin Neuropharmacol.* 1984;7(3):223-29.

67 Guttuso T Jr. Low-dose lithium adjunct therapy associated with reduced off-time in Parkinson's disease: a case series. *J Neurol Sci.* 2016;368:221-22.

68 Guttuso T Jr, Russak E, De Blanco MT, Ramanathan M. Could high lithium levels in tobacco contribute to reduced risk of Parkinson's disease in smokers? *J Neurol Sci.* 2019;397:179-80.

69 Pappas RS, Polzin GM, Zhang L, Watson CH, Paschal DC, Ashley DL. Cadmium, lead, and thallium in mainstream tobacco smoke particulate. *Food Chem Toxicol.* 2006;44(5):714-23;

    Wagner GJ, Yeargan R. Variation in cadmium accumulation potential and tissue distribution of cadmium in tobacco. *Plant Physiol.* 1986;82(1):274-79;

    Ashraf MW. Levels of heavy metals in popular cigarette brands and exposure to these metals via smoking. *ScientificWorldJournal.* 2012;2012:729430.

70 Yang Y, Ge Y, Zeng H, Zhou X, Peng L, Zeng Q. Phytoextraction of cadmium-contaminated soil and potential of regenerated tobacco biomass for recovery of cadmium. *Sci Rep.* 2017;7.

71 Guttuso T Jr, Russak E, De Blanco MT, Ramanathan M. Could high lithium levels in tobacco contribute to reduced risk of Parkinson's disease in smokers? *J Neurol Sci.* 2019;397:179-80;

    Ashraf MW. Levels of heavy metals in popular cigarette brands and exposure to these metals via smoking. *ScientificWorldJournal.* 2012;2012:729430.

72 Pappas RS, Fresquez MR, Martone N, Watson CH. Toxic metal concentrations in mainstream smoke from cigarettes available in the USA. *J Anal Toxicol.* 2014;38(4):204-11.

73 Richter P, Faroon O, Pappas RS. Cadmium and cadmium/zinc ratios and tobacco-related morbidities. *Int J Environ Res Public Health.* 2017;14(10):1154.

74 Adams SV, Newcomb PA. Cadmium blood and urine concentrations as measures of exposure: NHANES 1999-2010. *J Expo Sci Environ Epidemiol.* 2014;24(2):163-70;

    Mannino DM, Albalak R, Grosse S, Repace J. Second-hand smoke exposure and blood lead levels in U.S. children. *Epidemiology.* 2003;14(6):719-27;

    Li L, Guo L, Chen X, et al. Secondhand smoke is associated with heavy metal concentrations in children. *Eur J Pediatr.* 2018;177(2):257-64.

75 Nunes MA, Viel TA, Buck HS. Microdose lithium treatment stabilized cognitive impairment in patients with Alzheimer's disease. *Curr Alzheimer Res.* 2013;10(1):104-107.

76 Gallo V, Vineis P, Cancellieri M, et al. Exploring causality of the association between smoking and Parkinson's disease. *Int J Epidemiol.* 2018;48(3):912-25;

Liu W, Wang B, Xiao Y, Wang D, Chen W. Secondhand smoking and neurological disease: a meta-analysis of cohort studies. *Rev Environ Health.* 2020;36(2):271-77;

Guttuso T Jr, Russak E, De Blanco MT, Ramanathan M. Could high lithium levels in tobacco contribute to reduced risk of Parkinson's disease in smokers? *J Neurol Sci.* 2019;397:179-80.

77 Cataldo JK, Prochaska JJ, Glantz SA. Cigarette smoking is a risk factor for Alzheimer's disease: an analysis controlling for tobacco industry affiliation. *J Alzheimers Dis.* 2010;19(2):465-80.

78 Ghebremedhin E, Rosenberger A, Rüb U, et al. Inverse relationship between cerebrovascular lesions and severity of lewy body pathology in patients with lewy body diseases. *J Neuropathol Exp Neurol.* 2010;69(5):442-48.

79 Shorter E. The history of lithium therapy. *Bipolar Disord.* 2009;11(suppl 2):4-9.

80 Karimi A, Bahrampour K, Momeni Moghaddam MA, et al. Evaluation of lithium serum level in multiple sclerosis patients: a neuroprotective element. *Mult Scler Relat Disord.* 2017;17:244-48;

de Roos NM, de Vries JH, Katan MB. Serum lithium as a compliance marker for food and supplement intake. *Am J Clin Nutr.* 2001;73(1):75-79.

81 Guttuso T Jr, Russak E, De Blanco MT, Ramanathan M. Could high lithium levels in tobacco contribute to reduced risk of Parkinson's disease in smokers? *J Neurol Sci.* 2019;397:179-80.

82 Riedel S. Edward Jenner and the history of smallpox and vaccination. *Proc (Bayl Univ Med Cent).* 2005;18(1):21-25;

Miner J, Hoffhines A. The discovery of aspirin's antithrombotic effects. *Tex Heart Inst J.* 2007;34(2):179-86;

Lobanovska M, Pilla G. Penicillin's discovery and antibiotic resistance: lessons for the future? *Yale J Biol Med.* 2017;90(1):135-45.

83 Shorter E. The history of lithium therapy. *Bipolar Disord.* 2009;11(suppl 2):4-9.

84 Shorter E. The history of lithium therapy. *Bipolar Disord.* 2009;11(suppl 2):4-9.

85 Lähteenvuo M, Tanskanen A, Taipale H, et al. Real-world effectiveness of pharmacologic treatments for the prevention of rehospitalization in a Finnish nationwide cohort of patients with bipolar disorder. *JAMA Psychiatry.* 2018;75(4):347-55.

86 Manji HK, Moore GJ, Chen G. Lithium at 50: have the neuroprotective effects of this unique cation been overlooked? *Biol Psychiatry.* 1999;46(7):929-40.

87 Arraf Z, Amit T, Youdim MB, Farah R. Lithium and oxidative stress lessons from the MPTP model of Parkinson's disease. *Neurosci Lett.* 2012;516(1):57-61;

Kim YH, Rane A, Lussier S, Andersen JK. Lithium protects against oxidative stress-mediated cell death in alpha-synuclein-overexpressing in vitro and in vivo models of Parkinson's disease. *J Neurosci Res*. 2011;89(10):1666-75;

Lieu CA, Dewey CM, Chinta SJ, et al. Lithium prevents parkinsonian behavioral and striatal phenotypes in an aged parkin mutant transgenic mouse model. *Brain Res*. 2014;1591:111-177;

Nunes MA, Schöwe NM, Monteiro-Silva KC, et al. Chronic microdose lithium treatment prevented memory loss and neurohistopathological changes in a transgenic mouse model of Alzheimer's disease. *PLoS One*. 2015;10(11):e0142267;

Alural B, Ozerdem A, Allmer J, Genc K, Genc S. Lithium protects against paraquat neurotoxicity by NRF2 activation and miR-34a inhibition in SH-SY5Y cells. *Front Cell Neurosci*. 2015;9:209;

Chen RW, Chuang DM. Long term lithium treatment suppresses p53 and Bax expression but increases Bcl-2 expression. A prominent role in neuroprotection against excitotoxicity. *J Biol Chem*. 1999;274(10):6039-42;

Yu F, Wang Z, Tchantchou F, Chiu CT, Zhang Y, Chuang DM. Lithium ameliorates neurodegeneration, suppresses neuroinflammation, and improves behavioral performance in a mouse model of traumatic brain injury. *J Neurotrauma*. 2012;29(2):362-74;

Dong H, Zhang X, Dai X, et al. Lithium ameliorates lipopolysaccharide-induced microglial activation via inhibition of toll-like receptor 4 expression by activating the PI3K/Akt/FoxO1 pathway. *J Neuroinflammation*. 2014;11;

De-Paula VJ, Gattaz WF, Forlenza OV. Long-term lithium treatment increases intracellular and extracellular brain-derived neurotrophic factor (BDNF) in cortical and hippocampal neurons at subtherapeutic concentrations. *Bipolar Disord*. 2016;18(8):692-95;

Hou L, Xiong N, Liu L, et al. Lithium protects dopaminergic cells from rotenone toxicity via autophagy enhancement. *BMC Neurosci*. 2015;16(1);

Sarkar S, Floto RA, Berger Z, et al. Lithium induces autophagy by inhibiting inositol monophosphatase. *J Cell Biol*. 2005;170(7):1101-11;

Xiong N, Jia M, Chen C, et al. Potential autophagy enhancers attenuate rotenone-induced toxicity in SH-SY5Y. *Neuroscience*. 2011;199:292-302;

Jope RS. Lithium and GSK-3: one inhibitor, two inhibitory actions, multiple outcomes. *Trends Pharmacol Sci*. 2003;24(9):441-43;

Pan JQ, Lewis MC, Ketterman JK, et al. AKT kinase activity is required for lithium to modulate mood-related behaviors in mice. *Neuropsychopharmacology*. 2011;36(7):1397-411;

Struewing IT, Barnett CD, Tang T, Mao CD. Lithium increases PGC-1alpha expression and mitochondrial biogenesis in primary bovine aortic endothelial cells. *FEBS J*. 2007;274(11):2749-65;

Fornai F, Longone P, Ferrucci M, et al. Autophagy and amyotrophic lateral sclerosis: the multiple roles of lithium. *Autophagy.* 2008;4(4):527-30;

Shalbuyeva N, Brustovetsky T, Brustovetsky N. Lithium desensitizes brain mitochondria to calcium, antagonizes permeability transition, and diminishes cytochrome C release. *J Biol Chem.* 2007;282(25):18057-68;

Valvassori SS, Tonin PT, Varela RB, et al. Lithium modulates the production of peripheral and cerebral cytokines in an animal model of mania induced by dextroamphetamine. *Bipolar Disord.* 2015;17(5):507-17;

Zhao YJ, Qiao H, Liu DF, et al. Lithium promotes recovery after spinal cord injury. *Neural Regen Res.* 2022;17(6):1324-33.

88 Janka Z, Jones DG. Lithium entry into neural cells via sodium channels: a morphometric approach. *Neuroscience.* 1982;7(11):2849-57.

89 Thomas GA, Rhodes J, Green JT, Richardson C. Role of smoking in inflammatory bowel disease: implications for therapy. *Postgrad Med J.* 2000;76(895):273-79;

Zisook S. Ulcerative colitis: case responding to treatment with lithium carbonate. *JAMA* 1972;219(6):755;

Song F, Qureshi AA, Gao X, Li T, Han J. Smoking and risk of skin cancer: a prospective analysis and a meta-analysis. *Int J Epidemiol.* 2012;41(6):1694-705;

Odenbro A, Gillgren P, Bellocco R, Boffetta P, Håkansson N, Adami J. The risk for cutaneous malignant melanoma, melanoma in situ and intraocular malignant melanoma in relation to tobacco use and body mass index. *Br J Dermatol.* 2007;156(1):99-105;

Asgari MM, Chien AJ, Tsai AL, Fireman B, Quesenberry CP Jr. Association between lithium use and melanoma risk and mortality: a population-based study. *J Invest Dermatol.* 2017;137(10):2087-91.

90 Nunes MA, Schöwe NM, Monteiro-Silva KC, et al. Chronic microdose lithium treatment prevented memory loss and neurohistopathological changes in a transgenic mouse model of Alzheimer's disease. *PLoS One.* 2015;10(11):e0142267;

Leroy K, Ando K, Héraud C, et al. Lithium treatment arrests the development of neurofibrillary tangles in mutant tau transgenic mice with advanced neurofibrillary pathology. *J Alzheimers Dis.* 2010;19(2):705-19;

Noble W, Planel E, Zehr C, et al. Inhibition of glycogen synthase kinase-3 by lithium correlates with reduced tauopathy and degeneration in vivo. *Proc Natl Acad Sci U S A.* 2005;102(19):6990-95;

Zhang X, Heng X, Li T, et al. Long-term treatment with lithium alleviates memory deficits and reduces amyloid-beta production in an aged Alzheimer's disease transgenic mouse model. *J Alzheimers Dis.* 2011;24(4):739-49;

Fiorentini A, Rosi MC, Grossi C, Luccarini I, Casamenti F. Lithium improves hippocampal neurogenesis, neuropathology and cognitive functions in APP mutant mice. *PLoS One.* 2010;5(12):e14382.

91 Nunes MA, Schöwe NM, Monteiro-Silva KC, et al. Chronic microdose lithium treatment prevented memory loss and neurohistopathological changes in a transgenic mouse model of Alzheimer's disease. *PLoS One*. 2015;10(11):e0142267.

92 Arraf Z, Amit T, Youdim MB, Farah R. Lithium and oxidative stress lessons from the MPTP model of Parkinson's disease. *Neurosci Lett*. 2012;516(1):57-61;

Kim YH, Rane A, Lussier S, Andersen JK. Lithium protects against oxidative stress-mediated cell death in alpha-synuclein-overexpressing in vitro and in vivo models of Parkinson's disease. *J Neurosci Res*. 2011;89(10):1666-75;

Youdim MB, Arraf Z. Prevention of MPTP (N-methyl-4-phenyl-1,2,3,6-tetrahydropyridine) dopaminergic neurotoxicity in mice by chronic lithium: involvements of Bcl-2 and Bax. *Neuropharmacology*. 2004;46(8):1130-40.

93 Kim YH, Rane A, Lussier S, Andersen JK. Lithium protects against oxidative stress-mediated cell death in alpha-synuclein-overexpressing in vitro and in vivo models of Parkinson's disease. *J Neurosci Res*. 2011;89(10):1666-75;

Lieu CA, Dewey CM, Chinta SJ, et al. Lithium prevents parkinsonian behavioral and striatal phenotypes in an aged parkin mutant transgenic mouse model. *Brain Res*. 2014;1591:111-177.

94 Schrauzer GN. Lithium: occurrence, dietary intakes, nutritional essentiality. *J Am Coll Nutr*. 2002;21(4):14-21.

95 Kapusta ND, Mossaheb N, Etzersdorfer E, et al. Lithium in drinking water and suicide mortality. *Br J Psychiatry*. 2011;198(5):346-50.

96 Kapusta ND, Mossaheb N, Etzersdorfer E, et al. Lithium in drinking water and suicide mortality. *Br J Psychiatry*. 2011;198(5):346-50;

Schrauzer GN, Shrestha KP. Lithium in drinking water and the incidences of crimes, suicides, and arrests related to drug addictions. *Biol Trace Elem Res*. 1990;25(2):105-13;

Helbich M, Leitner M, Kapusta ND. Geospatial examination of lithium in drinking water and suicide mortality. *Int J Health Geogr*. 2012;11:19;

Ohgami H, Terao T, Shiotsuki I, Ishii N, Iwata N. Lithium levels in drinking water and risk of suicide. *Br J Psychiatry*. 2009;194(5):464-65; Dawson EB, Moore TD, McGanity WJ. Relationship of lithium metabolism to mental hospital admission and homicide. *Dis Nerv Syst*. 1972;33(8):546-56.

97 Knudsen NN, Schullehner J, Hansen B, et al. Lithium in drinking water and incidence of suicide: a nationwide individual-level cohort study with 22 years of follow-up. *Int J Environ Res Public Health*. 2017;14(6):627.

98 Zarse K, Terao T, Tian J, Iwata N, Ishii N, Ristow M. Low-dose lithium uptake promotes longevity in humans and metazoans. *Eur J Nutr*. 2011;50(5):387-89.

99 Voors AW. Lithium content of drinking water and ischemic heart disease. *N Engl J Med*. 1969;281(20):1132-33.

100 Kessing LV, Gerds TA, Knudsen NN, et al. Association of lithium in drinking water with the incidence of dementia. *JAMA Psychiatry*. 2017;74(10):1005-10.

101 Fajardo VA, Fajardo VA, LeBlanc PJ, MacPherson REK. Examining the relationship between trace lithium in drinking water and the rising rates of age-adjusted Alzheimer's disease mortality in Texas. *J Alzheimers Dis*. 2018;61(1):425-34.

102 Rossouw JE, Anderson GL, Prentice RL, et al. Risks and benefits of estrogen plus progestin in healthy postmenopausal women: principal results from the Women's Health Initiative randomized controlled trial. *Jama*. 2002;288(3):321-33.

103 Kessing LV, Nilsson FM. Increased risk of developing dementia in patients with major affective disorders compared to patients with other medical illnesses. *J Affect Disord*. 2003;73(3):261-69.

104 Nunes PV, Forlenza OV, Gattaz WF. Lithium and risk for Alzheimer's disease in elderly patients with bipolar disorder. *Br J Psychiatry*. 2007;190:359-60.

105 Kessing LV, Forman JL, Andersen PK. Does lithium protect against dementia? *Bipolar Disord*. 2010;12(1):87-94; Gerhard T, Devanand DP, Huang C, Crystal S, Olfson M. Lithium treatment and risk for dementia in adults with bipolar disorder: population-based cohort study. *Br J Psychiatry*. 2015;207(1):46-51.

106 Chen S, Underwood BR, Jones PB, Lewis JR, Cardinal RN. Association between lithium use and the incidence of dementia and its subtypes: a retrospective cohort study. *PLoS Med*. 2022;19(3):e1003941.

107 Chen S, Underwood BR, Jones PB, Lewis JR, Cardinal RN. Association between lithium use and the incidence of dementia and its subtypes: a retrospective cohort study. *PLoS Med*. 2022;19(3):e1003941.

108 Kessing LV, Gerds TA, Knudsen NN, et al. Association of lithium in drinking water with the incidence of dementia. *JAMA Psychiatry*. 2017;74(10):1005-10.

109 Kessing LV, Gerds TA, Knudsen NN, et al. Association of lithium in drinking water with the incidence of dementia. *JAMA Psychiatry*. 2017;74(10):1005-10.

110 Lan CC, Liu CC, Lin CH, et al. A reduced risk of stroke with lithium exposure in bipolar disorder: a population-based retrospective cohort study. *Bipolar Disord*. 2015;17(7):705-14;

Tsai SY, Shen RS, Kuo CJ, et al. The association between carotid atherosclerosis and treatment with lithium and antipsychotics in patients with bipolar disorder. *Aust N Z J Psychiatry*. 2020;54(11):1125-34.

111 Mohammadianinejad SE, Majdinasab N, Sajedi SA, Abdollahi F, Moqaddam MM, Sadr F. The effect of lithium in post-stroke motor recovery: a double-blind, placebo-controlled, randomized clinical trial. *Clin Neuropharmacol*. 2014;37(3):73-78.

112 Marras C, Herrmann N, Fischer HD, et al. Lithium use in older adults is associated with increased prescribing of Parkinson medications. *Am J Geriatr Psychiatry*. 2016;24(4):301-9.

113 Gelenberg AJ, Jefferson JW. Lithium tremor. *J Clin Psychiatry*. 1995;56(7):283-87.

114 Newman EJ, Breen K, Patterson J, Hadley DM, Grosset KA, Grosset DG. Accuracy of Parkinson's disease diagnosis in 610 general practice patients in the West of Scotland. *Mov Disord.* 2009;24(16):2379-85.

115 Marras C, Herrmann N, Fischer HD, et al. Lithium use in older adults is associated with increased prescribing of Parkinson medications. *Am J Geriatr Psychiatry.* 2016;24(4):301-9.

116 Forlenza OV, Diniz BS, Radanovic M, Santos FS, Talib LL, Gattaz WF. Disease-modifying properties of long-term lithium treatment for amnestic mild cognitive impairment: randomised controlled trial. *Br J Psychiatry.* 2011;198(5):351-56;

Wilkinson D, Holmes C, Woolford J, Stammers S, North J. Prophylactic therapy with lithium in elderly patients with unipolar major depression. *Int J Geriatr Psychiatry.* 2002;17(7):619-22.

117 Kessing LV, Forman JL, Andersen PK. Does lithium protect against dementia? *Bipolar Disord.* 2010;12(1):87-94;

Gerhard T, Devanand DP, Huang C, Crystal S, Olfson M. Lithium treatment and risk for dementia in adults with bipolar disorder: population-based cohort study. *Br J Psychiatry.* 2015;207(1):46-51;

Chen S, Underwood BR, Jones PB, Lewis JR, Cardinal RN. Association between lithium use and the incidence of dementia and its subtypes: a retrospective cohort study. *PLoS Med.* 2022;19(3):e1003941.

118 Ritz B, Ascherio A, Checkoway H, et al. Pooled analysis of tobacco use and risk of Parkinson disease. *Arch Neurol.* 2007;64(7):990-97;

Guttuso T Jr, Russak E, De Blanco MT, Ramanathan M. Could high lithium levels in tobacco contribute to reduced risk of Parkinson's disease in smokers? *J Neurol Sci.* 2019;397:179-80.

119 Kessing LV, Gerds TA, Knudsen NN, et al. Association of lithium in drinking water with the incidence of dementia. *JAMA Psychiatry.* 2017;74(10):1005-10.

120 Liu R, Gao X, Lu Y, Chen H. Meta-analysis of the relationship between Parkinson disease and melanoma. *Neurology.* 2011;76(23):2002-9;

Bertoni JM, Arlette JP, Fernandez HH, et al. Increased melanoma risk in Parkinson disease: a prospective clinicopathological study. *Arch Neurol.* 2010;67(3):347-52.

121 Gao X, Simon KC, Han J, Schwarzschild MA, Ascherio A. Family history of melanoma and Parkinson disease risk. *Neurology.* 2009;73(16):1286-91;

Olsen JH, Friis S, Frederiksen K. Malignant melanoma and other types of cancer preceding Parkinson disease. *Epidemiology.* 2006;17(5):582-87.

122 Song F, Qureshi AA, Gao X, Li T, Han J. Smoking and risk of skin cancer: a prospective analysis and a meta-analysis. *Int J Epidemiol.* 2012;41(6):1694-705;

Odenbro A, Gillgren P, Bellocco R, Boffetta P, Håkansson N, Adami J. The risk for cutaneous malignant melanoma, melanoma in situ and intraocular malignant melanoma in relation to tobacco use and body mass index. *Br J Dermatol.* 2007;156(1):99-105.

123 Guttuso T Jr, Russak E, De Blanco MT, Ramanathan M. Could high lithium levels in tobacco contribute to reduced risk of Parkinson's disease in smokers? *J Neurol Sci.* 2019;397:179-80.

124 Guttuso T Jr. High lithium levels in tobacco may account for reduced incidences of both Parkinson's disease and melanoma in smokers through enhanced β-catenin-mediated activity. *Med Hypotheses.* 2019;131:109302.

125 Berwick DC, Harvey K. The importance of Wnt signalling for neurodegeneration in Parkinson's disease. *Biochem Soc Trans.* 2012;40(5):1123-28.

126 Decressac M, Volakakis N, Björklund A, Perlmann T. NURR1 in Parkinson disease—from pathogenesis to therapeutic potential. *Nat Rev Neurol.* 2013;9(11):629-36.

127 Li T, Yang Z, Li S, Cheng C, Shen B, Le W. Alterations of NURR1 and cytokines in the peripheral blood mononuclear cells: combined biomarkers for Parkinson's disease. *Front Aging Neurosci.* 2018;10:392;

Chu Y, Le W, Kompoliti K, Jankovic J, Mufson EJ, Kordower JH. Nurr1 in Parkinson's disease and related disorders. *J Comp Neurol.* 2006;494(3):495-514.

128 Chu Y, Kompoliti K, Cochran EJ, Mufson EJ, Kordower JH. Age-related decreases in Nurr1 immunoreactivity in the human substantia nigra. *J Comp Neurol.* 2002;450(3):203-14;

Berwick DC, Javaheri B, Wetzel A, et al. Pathogenic *LRRK2* variants are gain-of-function mutations that enhance LRRK2-mediated repression of β-catenin signaling. *Mol Neurodegener.* 2017;12(1):9;

Awad O, Panicker LM, Deranieh RM, et al. Altered differentiation potential of Gaucher's disease iPSC neuronal progenitors due to Wnt/β-catenin downregulation. *Stem Cell Reports.* 2017;9(6):1853-67.

129 Zhang L, Cen L, Qu S, et al. Enhancing beta-catenin activity via GSK3beta inhibition protects PC12 cells against rotenone toxicity through Nurr1 induction. *PLoS One* 2016;11(4):e0152931.

130 Chien AJ, Moore EC, Lonsdorf AS, et al. Activated Wnt/β-catenin signaling in melanoma is associated with decreased proliferation in patient tumors and a murine melanoma model. *Proc Natl Acad Sci U S A.* 2009;106(4):1193-98.

131 Asgari MM, Chien AJ, Tsai AL, Fireman B, Quesenberry CP Jr. Association between lithium use and melanoma risk and mortality: a population-based study. *J Invest Dermatol.* 2017;137(10):2087-91.

132 Pan T, Li X, Jankovic J. The association between Parkinson's disease and melanoma. *Int J Cancer.* 2011;128(10):2251-60;

Bajaj A, Driver JA, Schernhammer ES. Parkinson's disease and cancer risk: a systematic review and meta-analysis. *Cancer Causes Control.* 2010;21(5):697-707.

133   Giles RH, van Es JH, Clevers H. Caught up in a Wnt storm: Wnt signaling in cancer. *Biochim Biophys Acta.* 2003;1653(1):1-24.

134   Zhang L, Cen L, Qu S, et al. Enhancing beta-catenin activity via GSK3beta inhibition protects PC12 cells against rotenone toxicity through Nurr1 induction. *PLoS One* 2016;11(4):e0152931.

135   Martinsson L, Westman J, Hällgren J, Ösby U, Backlund L. Lithium treatment and cancer incidence in bipolar disorder. *Bipolar Disord.* 2016;18(1):33-40;

      Huang RY, Hsieh KP, Huang WW, Yang YH. Use of lithium and cancer risk in patients with bipolar disorder: population-based cohort study. *Br J Psychiatry.* 2016;209(5):393-99.

136   Coffey CE, Ross DR, Ferren EL, Sullivan JL, Olanow CW. Treatment of the "on-off" phenomenon in Parkinsonism with lithium carbonate. *Ann Neurol.* 1982;12:375-79.

137   Coffey CE, Ross DR, Massey EW, Olanow CW. Dyskinesias associated with lithium therapy in parkinsonism. *Clin Neuropharmacol.* 1984;7(3):223-29.

138   Guttuso T Jr. Low-dose lithium adjunct therapy associated with reduced off-time in Parkinson's disease: a case series. *J Neurol Sci.* 2016;368:221-22.

139   Macdonald A, Briggs K, Poppe M, Higgins A, Velayudhan L, Lovestone S. A feasibility and tolerability study of lithium in Alzheimer's disease. *Int J Geriatr Psychiatry.* 2008;23(7):704-11.

140   Hampel H, Ewers M, Bürger K, et al. Lithium trial in Alzheimer's disease: a randomized, single-blind, placebo-controlled, multicenter 10-week study. *J Clin Psychiatry.* 2009;70(6):922-31.

141   Tabert MH, Manly JJ, Liu X, et al. Neuropsychological prediction of conversion to Alzheimer disease in patients with mild cognitive impairment. *Arch Gen Psychiatry.* 2006;63(8):916-24.

142   Forlenza OV, Diniz BS, Radanovic M, Santos FS, Talib LL, Gattaz WF. Disease-modifying properties of long-term lithium treatment for amnestic mild cognitive impairment: randomised controlled trial. *Br J Psychiatry.* 2011;198(5):351-56.

143   Moscoso A, Grothe MJ, Ashton NJ, et al. Longitudinal associations of blood phosphorylated tau181 and neurofilament light chain with neurodegeneration in Alzheimer disease. *JAMA Neurol.* 2021;78(4):396-406;

      Karikari TK, Pascoal TA, Ashton NJ, et al. Blood phosphorylated tau 181 as a biomarker for Alzheimer's disease: a diagnostic performance and prediction modelling study using data from four prospective cohorts. *Lancet Neurol.* 2020;19(5):422-33.

144   Forlenza OV, Radanovic M, Talib LL, Gattaz WF. Clinical and biological effects of long-term lithium treatment in older adults with amnestic mild cognitive impairment: randomised clinical trial. *Br J Psychiatry.* 2019;215(5):668-74.

145   Nunes MA, Viel TA, Buck HS. Microdose lithium treatment stabilized

cognitive impairment in patients with Alzheimer's disease. *Curr Alzheimer Res.* 2013;10(1):104-107.

146 Nunes MA, Viel TA, Buck HS. Microdose lithium treatment stabilized cognitive impairment in patients with Alzheimer's disease. *Curr Alzheimer Res.* 2013;10(1):104-107.

147 Nunes MA, Viel TA, Buck HS. Microdose lithium treatment stabilized cognitive impairment in patients with Alzheimer's disease. *Curr Alzheimer Res.* 2013;10(1):104-107.

148 Chen S, Underwood BR, Jones PB, Lewis JR, Cardinal RN. Association between lithium use and the incidence of dementia and its subtypes: A retrospective cohort study. *PLoS Med* 2022;19:e1003941.

149 Guttuso T Jr. High lithium levels in tobacco may account for reduced incidences of both Parkinson's disease and melanoma in smokers through enhanced β-catenin-mediated activity. *Med Hypotheses.* 2019;131:109302.

150 Bown SR. Scurvy: *How a Surgeon, a Mariner, and a Gentlemen Solved the Greatest Medical Mystery of the Age of Sail.* Thomas Dunne Books; 2003.

151 Durzan DJ. Arginine, scurvy and Cartier's "tree of life." *J Ethnobiol Ethnomed.* 2009;5.

152 Durzan DJ. Arginine, scurvy and Cartier's "tree of life." *J Ethnobiol Ethnomed.* 2009;5.

153 Bown SR. Scurvy: *How a Surgeon, a Mariner, and a Gentlemen Solved the Greatest Medical Mystery of the Age of Sail.* Thomas Dunne Books; 2003.

154 Wikipedia. George Anson's voyage around the world. Updated August 17, 2022. Accessed September 19, 2022. https://en.wikipedia.org/wiki/George_Anson%27s_voyage_around_the_world.

155 Lind J. *A treatise of the scurvy, in three parts. Containing an inquiry into the nature, causes, and cure, of that disease. Together with a critical and chronological view of what has been published on the subject.* Sands, Murray and Cochran; 1753. https://archive.org/details/b30507054/page/190/mode/2up.

156 Lind J. *A treatise of the scurvy, in three parts. Containing an inquiry into the nature, causes, and cure, of that disease. Together with a critical and chronological view of what has been published on the subject.* Sands, Murray and Cochran; 1753. https://archive.org/details/b30507054/page/190/mode/2up.

157 Bown SR. Scurvy: *How a Surgeon, a Mariner, and a Gentlemen Solved the Greatest Medical Mystery of the Age of Sail.* Thomas Dunne Books; 2003.

158 Bartholomew M. James Lind and scurvy: a revaluation. *J Marit Res.* 2002;4(1):1-14.

159 Riedel S. Edward Jenner and the history of smallpox and vaccination. *Proc (Bayl Univ Med Cent).* 2005;18(1):21-25; Lobanovska M, Pilla G. Penicillin's discovery and antibiotic resistance: lessons for the future? *Yale J Biol Med.* 2017;90(1):135-45.

160 Macdonald A, Briggs K, Poppe M, Higgins A, Velayudhan L, Lovestone S. A

feasibility and tolerability study of lithium in Alzheimer's disease. *Int J Geriatr Psychiatry*. 2008;23(7):704-11;

Hampel H, Ewers M, Bürger K, et al. Lithium trial in Alzheimer's disease: a randomized, single-blind, placebo-controlled, multicenter 10-week study. *J Clin Psychiatry*. 2009;70(6):922-31.

161 Galpern WR. NINDS pilot therapeutics network investigators: lithium in progressive supranuclear palsy and corticobasal degeneration. *Mov Disord*. 2010;25(suppl 2):S498.

162 Macdonald A, Briggs K, Poppe M, Higgins A, Velayudhan L, Lovestone S. A feasibility and tolerability study of lithium in Alzheimer's disease. *Int J Geriatr Psychiatry*. 2008;23(7):704-11.

163 Nunes MA, Viel TA, Buck HS. Microdose lithium treatment stabilized cognitive impairment in patients with Alzheimer's disease. *Curr Alzheimer Res*. 2013;10(1):104-107;

Forlenza OV, Diniz BS, Radanovic M, Santos FS, Talib LL, Gattaz WF. Disease-modifying properties of long-term lithium treatment for amnestic mild cognitive impairment: randomised controlled trial. *Br J Psychiatry*. 2011;198(5):351-56;

Forlenza OV, Radanovic M, Talib LL, Gattaz WF. Clinical and biological effects of long-term lithium treatment in older adults with amnestic mild cognitive impairment: randomised clinical trial. *Br J Psychiatry*. 2019;215(5):668-74.

164 Saccà F, Marsili A, Quarantelli M, et al. A randomized clinical trial of lithium in multiple system atrophy. *J Neurol*. 2013;260(2):458-61.

165 Guttuso T Jr. Low-dose lithium adjunct therapy associated with reduced off-time in Parkinson's disease: a case series. *J Neurol Sci*. 2016;368:221-22;

Nunes MA, Viel TA, Buck HS. Microdose lithium treatment stabilized cognitive impairment in patients with Alzheimer's disease. *Curr Alzheimer Res*. 2013;10(1):104-107;

Forlenza OV, Diniz BS, Radanovic M, Santos FS, Talib LL, Gattaz WF. Disease-modifying properties of long-term lithium treatment for amnestic mild cognitive impairment: randomised controlled trial. *Br J Psychiatry*. 2011;198(5):351-56;

Macdonald A, Briggs K, Poppe M, Higgins A, Velayudhan L, Lovestone S. A feasibility and tolerability study of lithium in Alzheimer's disease. *Int J Geriatr Psychiatry*. 2008;23(7):704-11;

Forlenza OV, Radanovic M, Talib LL, Gattaz WF. Clinical and biological effects of long-term lithium treatment in older adults with amnestic mild cognitive impairment: randomised clinical trial. *Br J Psychiatry*. 2019;215(5):668-74.

166 Gildengers A. Lithium as a treatment to prevent impairment of cognition in elders (LATTICE). Updated June 7, 2022. Accessed September 19, 2022. https://clinicaltrials.gov/ct2/show/NCT03185208?term=lithium&recrs=ab&cond=Alzheimer+Disease&draw=2&rank=1.

167 Shorter E. The history of lithium therapy. *Bipolar Disord*. 2009;11(suppl 2):4-9.

168 Johnston AM, Eagles JM. Lithium-associated clinical hypothyroidism. Prevalence and risk factors. *Br J Psychiatry.* 1999;175:336-39;

Aiff H, Attman PO, Aurell M, et al. Effects of 10 to 30 years of lithium treatment on kidney function. *J Psychopharmacol.* 2015;29(5):608-14.

169 Aprahamian I, Santos FS, dos Santos B, et al. Long-term, low-dose lithium treatment does not impair renal function in the elderly: a 2-year randomized, placebo-controlled trial followed by single-blind extension. *J Clin Psychiatry.* 2014;75(7):e672-78.

170 Guttuso T Jr, Kurlan R, McDermott MP, Kieburtz K. Gabapentin's effects on hot flashes in postmenopausal women: a randomized controlled trial. *Obstet Gynecol.* 2003;101(2):337-45.

171 Nunes MA, Viel TA, Buck HS. Microdose lithium treatment stabilized cognitive impairment in patients with Alzheimer's disease. *Curr Alzheimer Res.* 2013;10(1):104-107;

Forlenza OV, Diniz BS, Radanovic M, Santos FS, Talib LL, Gattaz WF. Disease-modifying properties of long-term lithium treatment for amnestic mild cognitive impairment: randomised controlled trial. *Br J Psychiatry* 2011;198:351-6;

Forlenza OV, Radanovic M, Talib LL, Gattaz WF. Clinical and biological effects of long-term lithium treatment in older adults with amnestic mild cognitive impairment: randomised clinical trial. *Br J Psychiatry.* 2019;215(5):668-74.

172 Greenblatt J. *Integrative Medicine for Alzheimer's: The Breakthrough Natural Treatment Plan that Prevents Alzheimer's Using Nutritional Lithium.* FriesenPress; 2018;

Greenblatt J, Grossmann K. *Nutritional Lithium: A Cinderella Story: The Untold Tale of a Mineral That Transforms Lives and Heals the Brain.* CreateSpace Independent Publishing Platform; 2016.

173 Sabuncu MR, Desikan RS, Sepulcre J, et al. The dynamics of cortical and hippocampal atrophy in Alzheimer disease. *Arch Neurol.* 2011;68(8):1040-48.

174 Ofori E, DeKosky ST, Febo M, et al. Free-water imaging of the hippocampus is a sensitive marker of Alzheimer's disease. *Neuroimage Clin.* 2019;24:101985.

175 Febo M, Perez PD, Ceballos-Diaz C, et al. Diffusion magnetic resonance imaging-derived free water detects neurodegenerative pattern induced by interferon-γ. *Brain Struct Funct.* 2020;225(1):427-39;

Pasternak O, Shenton ME, Westin CF. Estimation of extracellular volume from regularized multi-shell diffusion MRI. *Med Image Comput Comput Assist Interv.* 2012;15(pt 2):305-12.

176 Burciu RG, Ofori E, Archer DB, et al. Progression marker of Parkinson's disease: a 4-year multisite imaging study. *Brain.* 2017;140(8):2183-92;

Guttuso T Jr, Sirica D, Tosun D, et al. Thalamic dorsomedial nucleus free water correlates with cognitive decline in Parkinson's disease. *Mov Disord.* 2022;37(3):490-501.

177 Bearden CE, Thompson PM, Dutton RA, et al. Three-dimensional mapping of

hippocampal anatomy in unmedicated and lithium-treated patients with bipolar disorder. *Neuropsychopharmacology.* 2008;33(6):1229-38;

Beyer JL, Kuchibhatla M, Payne ME, et al. Hippocampal volume measurement in older adults with bipolar disorder. *Am J Geriatr Psychiatry.* 2004;12(6):613-20;

Simonetti A, Sani G, Dacquino C, et al. Hippocampal subfield volumes in short- and long-term lithium-treated patients with bipolar I disorder. *Bipolar Disord.* 2016;18(4):352-62;

van Erp TG, Thompson PM, Kieseppä T, et al. Hippocampal morphology in lithium and non-lithium-treated bipolar I disorder patients, non-bipolar co-twins, and control twins. *Hum Brain Mapp.* 2012;33(3):501-10;

Yucel K, Taylor VH, McKinnon MC, et al. Bilateral hippocampal volume increase in patients with bipolar disorder and short-term lithium treatment. *Neuropsychopharmacology.* 2008;33(2):361-67.

178 Nunes MA, Viel TA, Buck HS. Microdose lithium treatment stabilized cognitive impairment in patients with Alzheimer's disease. *Curr Alzheimer Res.* 2013;10(1):104-107;

Forlenza OV, Diniz BS, Radanovic M, Santos FS, Talib LL, Gattaz WF. Disease-modifying properties of long-term lithium treatment for amnestic mild cognitive impairment: randomised controlled trial. *Br J Psychiatry.* 2011;198(5):351-56;

Forlenza OV, Radanovic M, Talib LL, Gattaz WF. Clinical and biological effects of long-term lithium treatment in older adults with amnestic mild cognitive impairment: randomised clinical trial. *Br J Psychiatry.* 2019;215(5):668-74.

179 Gildengers A. Lithium as a treatment to prevent impairment of cognition in elders (LATTICE). Updated June 7, 2022. Accessed September 19, 2022. https://clinicaltrials.gov/ct2/show/NCT03185208?term=lithium&recrs= ab&cond=Alzheimer+Disease&draw=2&rank=1.

180 Bearden CE, Thompson PM, Dutton RA, et al. Three-dimensional mapping of hippocampal anatomy in unmedicated and lithium-treated patients with bipolar disorder. *Neuropsychopharmacology.* 2008;33(6):1229-38;

Beyer JL, Kuchibhatla M, Payne ME, et al. Hippocampal volume measurement in older adults with bipolar disorder. *Am J Geriatr Psychiatry.* 2004;12(6):613-20;

Simonetti A, Sani G, Dacquino C, et al. Hippocampal subfield volumes in short- and long-term lithium-treated patients with bipolar I disorder. *Bipolar Disord.* 2016;18(4):352-62;

van Erp TG, Thompson PM, Kieseppä T, et al. Hippocampal morphology in lithium and non-lithium-treated bipolar I disorder patients, non-bipolar co-twins, and control twins. *Hum Brain Mapp.* 2012;33(3):501-10;

Yucel K, Taylor VH, McKinnon MC, et al. Bilateral hippocampal volume increase in patients with bipolar disorder and short-term lithium treatment. *Neuropsychopharmacology.* 2008;33(2):361-67.

181 Moore GJ, Cortese BM, Glitz DA, et al. A longitudinal study of the effects

of lithium treatment on prefrontal and subgenual prefrontal gray matter volume in treatment-responsive bipolar disorder patients. *J Clin Psychiatry.* 2009;70(5):699-705;

Gildengers AG, Butters MA, Aizenstein HJ, et al. Longer lithium exposure is associated with better white matter integrity in older adults with bipolar disorder. *Bipolar Disord.* 2015;17(3):248-56;

Haarman BCM, Riemersma-Van der Lek RF, Burger H, et al. Diffusion tensor imaging in euthymic bipolar disorder—a tract-based spatial statistics study. *J Affect Disord.* 2016;203:281-91;

Hajek T, Bauer M, Pfennig A, et al. Large positive effect of lithium on prefrontal cortex N-acetylaspartate in patients with bipolar disorder: 2-centre study. *J Psychiatry Neurosci.* 2012;37(3):185-92;

Sassi RB, Brambilla P, Hatch JP, et al. Reduced left anterior cingulate volumes in untreated bipolar patients. *Biol Psychiatry.* 2004;56(7):467-75.

182 Forlenza OV, Diniz BS, Radanovic M, Santos FS, Talib LL, Gattaz WF. Disease-modifying properties of long-term lithium treatment for amnestic mild cognitive impairment: randomised controlled trial. *Br J Psychiatry.* 2011;198(5):351-56.

183 Guttuso T Jr. Low-dose lithium adjunct therapy associated with reduced off-time in Parkinson's disease: a case series. *J Neurol Sci.* 2016;368:221-22.

184 van Heerden JH, Conesa A, Stein DJ, Montaner D, Russell V, Illing N. Parallel changes in gene expression in peripheral blood mononuclear cells and the brain after maternal separation in the mouse. *BMC Res Notes.* 2009;2:195.

185 Lin CH, Yang SY, Horng HE, et al. Plasma α-synuclein predicts cognitive decline in Parkinson's disease. *J Neurol Neurosurg Psychiatry.* 2017;88(10):818-24.

186 Le W, Conneely OM, He Y, Jankovic J, Appel SH. Reduced Nurr1 expression increases the vulnerability of mesencephalic dopamine neurons to MPTP-induced injury. *J Neurochem.* 1999;73(5):2218-21;

Decressac M, Kadkhodaei B, Mattsson B, Laguna A, Perlmann T, Björklund A. α-Synuclein-induced down-regulation of Nurr1 disrupts GDNF signaling in nigral dopamine neurons. *Sci Transl Med.* 2012;4(163):163ra156.

187 Chu Y, Kompoliti K, Cochran EJ, Mufson EJ, Kordower JH. Age-related decreases in Nurr1 immunoreactivity in the human substantia nigra. *J Comp Neurol.* 2002;450(3):203-14.

188 Li T, Yang Z, Li S, Cheng C, Shen B, Le W. Alterations of NURR1 and cytokines in the peripheral blood mononuclear cells: combined biomarkers for Parkinson's disease. *Front Aging Neurosci.* 2018;10:392;

Chu Y, Le W, Kompoliti K, Jankovic J, Mufson EJ, Kordower JH. Nurr1 in Parkinson's disease and related disorders. *J Comp Neurol.* 2006;494(3):495-514.

189 Saijo K, Winner B, Carson CT, et al. A Nurr1/CoREST pathway in microglia and astrocytes protects dopaminergic neurons from inflammation-induced death. *Cell.* 2009;137(1):47-59;

Yang YX, Latchman DS. Nurr1 transcriptionally regulates the expression of alpha-synuclein. *Neuroreport.* 2008;19(8):867-71.

190 Zhang L, Cen L, Qu S, et al. Enhancing beta-catenin activity via GSK3beta inhibition protects PC12 cells against rotenone toxicity through Nurr1 induction. *PLoS One* 2016;11(4):e0152931.

191 Zetterström RH, Williams R, Perlmann T, Olson L. Cellular expression of the immediate early transcription factors Nurr1 and NGFI-B suggests a gene regulatory role in several brain regions including the nigrostriatal dopamine system. *Brain Res Mol Brain Res.* 1996;41(1-2):111-20;

Lin X, Parisiadou L, Sgobio C, et al. Conditional expression of Parkinson's disease-related mutant α-synuclein in the midbrain dopaminergic neurons causes progressive neurodegeneration and degradation of transcription factor nuclear receptor related 1. *J Neurosci.* 2012;32(27):9248-64;

Jeon SG, Yoo A, Chun DW, et al. The critical role of Nurr1 as a mediator and therapeutic target in Alzheimer's disease-related pathogenesis. *Aging Dis.* 2020;11(3):705-24.

192 Zhang L, Cen L, Qu S, et al. Enhancing Beta-Catenin Activity via GSK3beta Inhibition Protects PC12 Cells against Rotenone Toxicity through Nurr1 Induction. *PLoS One* 2016;11:e0152931.

193 Febo M, Perez PD, Ceballos-Diaz C, et al. Diffusion magnetic resonance imaging-derived free water detects neurodegenerative pattern induced by interferon-γ. *Brain Struct Funct.* 2020;225(1):427-39;

Pasternak O, Shenton ME, Westin CF. Estimation of extracellular volume from regularized multi-shell diffusion MRI. *Med Image Comput Comput Assist Interv.* 2012;15(pt 2):305-12;

Burciu RG, Ofori E, Archer DB, et al. Progression marker of Parkinson's disease: a 4-year multisite imaging study. *Brain.* 2017;140(8):2183-92;

Guttuso T Jr, Sirica D, Tosun D, et al. Thalamic dorsomedial nucleus free water correlates with cognitive decline in Parkinson's disease. *Mov Disord.* 2022;37(3):490-501.

194 Burciu RG, Ofori E, Archer DB, et al. Progression marker of Parkinson's disease: a 4-year multisite imaging study. *Brain.* 2017;140(8):2183-92.

195 Guttuso T Jr, Sirica D, Tosun D, et al. Thalamic dorsomedial nucleus free water correlates with cognitive decline in Parkinson's disease. *Mov Disord.* 2022;37(3):490-501.

196 Burciu RG, Ofori E, Archer DB, et al. Progression marker of Parkinson's disease: a 4-year multisite imaging study. *Brain.* 2017;140(8):2183-92;

Guttuso T Jr, Sirica D, Tosun D, et al. Thalamic dorsomedial nucleus free water correlates with cognitive decline in Parkinson's disease. *Mov Disord.* 2022;37(3):490-501.

197 Febo M, Perez PD, Ceballos-Diaz C, et al. Diffusion magnetic resonance imaging-derived free water detects neurodegenerative pattern induced by interferon-γ. *Brain Struct Funct.* 2020;225(1):427-39;

Pasternak O, Shenton ME, Westin CF. Estimation of extracellular volume from regularized multi-shell diffusion MRI. *Med Image Comput Comput Assist Interv.* 2012;15(pt 2):305-12.

198 Gildengers A. Lithium as a treatment to prevent impairment of cognition in elders (LATTICE). Updated June 7, 2022. Accessed September 19, 2022. https://clinicaltrials.gov/ct2/show/NCT03185208?term=lithium&recrs=ab&cond=Alzheimer+Disease&draw=2&rank=1.

199 Dintica CS, Marseglia A, Rizzuto D, et al. Impaired olfaction is associated with cognitive decline and neurodegeneration in the brain. *Neurology.* 2019;92(7):e700-e709;

Sensonics International. Brief Smell Identification Test (BSIT). Accessed September 20, 2022. https://sensonics.com/product/brief-smell-identification-test-b-sit-version-cross-cultural-smell-identification-test/.

200 Sensonics International. Brief Smell Identification Test (BSIT). Accessed September 20, 2022. https://sensonics.com/product/brief-smell-identification-test-b-sit-version-cross-cultural-smell-identification-test/.

201 Aiff H, Attman PO, Aurell M, et al. Effects of 10 to 30 years of lithium treatment on kidney function. *J Psychopharmacol.* 2015;29(5):608-14;

Aprahamian I, Santos FS, dos Santos B, et al. Long-term, low-dose lithium treatment does not impair renal function in the elderly: a 2-year randomized, placebo-controlled trial followed by single-blind extension. *J Clin Psychiatry.* 2014;75(7):e672-78.

202 Johnston AM, Eagles JM. Lithium-associated clinical hypothyroidism. Prevalence and risk factors. *Br J Psychiatry* 1999;175:336-9;

Aiff H, Attman PO, Aurell M, et al. Effects of 10 to 30 years of lithium treatment on kidney function. *J Psychopharmacol* 2015;29:608-14.

203 Aprahamian I, Santos FS, dos Santos B, et al. Long-term, low-dose lithium treatment does not impair renal function in the elderly: a 2-year randomized, placebo-controlled trial followed by single-blind extension. *J Clin Psychiatry* 2014;75:e672-8.

204 Janka Z, Jones DG. Lithium entry into neural cells via sodium channels: a morphometric approach. *Neuroscience.* 1982;7(11):2849-57.

205 Smith DF. Lithium orotate, carbonate and chloride: pharmacokinetics, polyuria in rats. *Br J Pharmacol.* 1976;56(4):399-402.

206 Kling MA, Manowitz P, Pollack IW. Rat brain and serum lithium concentrations after acute injections of lithium carbonate and orotate. *J Pharm Pharmacol.* 1978;30(6):368-70.

207 Laconi E, Denda A, Rao PM, Rajalakshmi S, Pani P, Sarma DS. Studies on liver tumor promotion in the rat by orotic acid: dose and minimum exposure time required for dietary orotic acid to promote hepatocarcinogenesis. *Carcinogenesis*. 1993;14(9):1771-75;

Laconi E, Vasudevan S, Rao PM, Rajalakshmi S, Pani P, Sarma DS. The effect of long-term feeding of orotic acid on the incidence of foci of enzyme-altered hepatocytes and hepatic nodules in Fischer 344 rats. *Carcinogenesis*. 1993;14(9):1901-5.

208 Centers for Disease Control and Prevention. Health effects of secondhand smoke. Updated June 14, 2021. Accessed September 20, 2022. https://www.cdc.gov/tobacco/data_statistics/fact_sheets/secondhand_smoke/health_effects/index.htm.

209 Leaf Group Ltd. Lithium aspartate vs. lithium orotate. LEAFtv. Accessed September 20, 2022. https://www.leaf.tv/articles/lithium-aspartate-vs-lithium-orotate/.

210 Park CH, Choi SH, Piao Y, et al. Glutamate and aspartate impair memory retention and damage hypothalamic neurons in adult mice. *Toxicol Lett*. 2000;115(2):117-25.

211 Kessing LV, Gerds TA, Knudsen NN, et al. Association of lithium in drinking water with the incidence of dementia. *JAMA Psychiatry*. 2017;74(10):1005-10.

212 Nunes MA, Viel TA, Buck HS. Microdose lithium treatment stabilized cognitive impairment in patients with Alzheimer's disease. *Curr Alzheimer Res*. 2013;10(1):104-107.

213 Ritz B, Ascherio A, Checkoway H, et al. Pooled analysis of tobacco use and risk of Parkinson disease. *Arch Neurol*. 2007;64(7):990-97;

Guttuso T Jr, Russak E, De Blanco MT, Ramanathan M. Could high lithium levels in tobacco contribute to reduced risk of Parkinson's disease in smokers? *J Neurol Sci*. 2019;397:179-80.

214 Forlenza OV, Diniz BS, Radanovic M, Santos FS, Talib LL, Gattaz WF. Disease-modifying properties of long-term lithium treatment for amnestic mild cognitive impairment: randomised controlled trial. *Br J Psychiatry*. 2011;198(5):351-56.

215 Chen S, Underwood BR, Jones PB, Lewis JR, Cardinal RN. Association between lithium use and the incidence of dementia and its subtypes: a retrospective cohort study. *PLoS Med*. 2022;19(3):e1003941.

216 Nunes MA, Viel TA, Buck HS. Microdose lithium treatment stabilized cognitive impairment in patients with Alzheimer's disease. *Curr Alzheimer Res*. 2013;10(1):104-107.

217 Gildengers A. Lithium as a treatment to prevent impairment of cognition in elders (LATTICE). Updated June 7, 2022. Accessed September 19, 2022. https://clinicaltrials.gov/ct2/show/NCT03185208?term=lithium&recrs=ab&cond=Alzheimer+Disease&draw=2&rank=1.

Made in the USA
Columbia, SC
16 May 2023

16804453R00102